~ Reiki Touch ~

For Nurses

Healing Through the Energy System

An incredible method of energy healing that joins the nurse and patient at the heart level

By Debbie Glasgow RN,CRMI,CHTP
Certified Reiki Touch Instructor

ISBN-13 978-1-60145-275-7

ISBN-10 1-60145-275-6

The International Center for Reiki Touch Training

c/o Debbie Glasgow RN

4990 Tawas Dr.

Ottawa Lake, Mi. 49267

www.ReikiTouch.us

Reikiceu@aol.com

Dedicated to all of the nurses and nursing students of America. You are very important in the lives of many who suffer and are in need of your compassionate care and guidance.

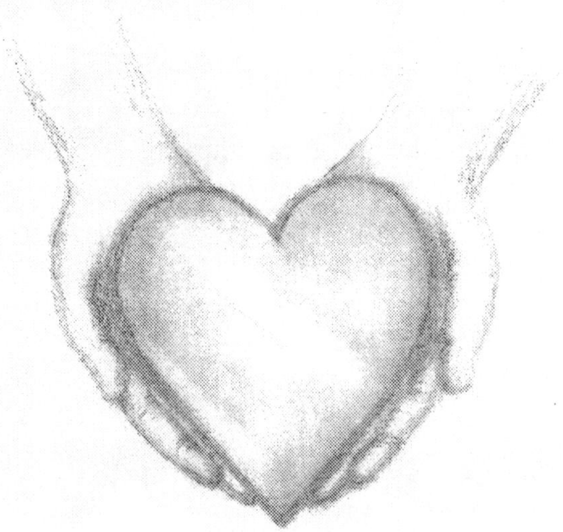

Heart in Hands Drawing by Barb Kenner RN

Table of Contents

Note to Readers:

The Reiki Touch concepts and techniques taught in this book are not intended as a substitute for surgical or medical treatment. The Reiki Touch therapy is used as a complimentary tool for holistic healing of mind, body, emotion, and spirit collectively.

Acknowledgements

I Honor and thank my Great Grandmother, and Cherokee ancestor, Vicy Williamson-Monday, for all the knowledge and values she left behind. Her energy and wisdom sustains itself today in many ways, such as in the manifestation of this book, including the messages about life and the value of healing brought through it.

I acknowledge and give deep thanks to my parents Herbert and Veronica Moore for helping me be aware of my inner strength, which is the tool that guides me in writing this book. I also give thanks to my grandparents, Walter and Hattie Moore, Raymond and Leona Diroff who taught me to love myself and to honor and respect all people of the world in a way that I would like to be loved, honored and respected.

Words cannot express the deep thankfulness I have for my husband, Rev. Steven, who has helped me above and beyond what was ever expected. He was always there helping with editing, gathering information and emotional support. He and my daughter, Richelle Reynolds, were both a great inspiration for many of the techniques taught in the Reiki Touch program as well as a reminder of the depth of healing that can occur with the Reiki energy, which further moved me to write this book.

I give special thanks to my friend Dr. Steven Gaynor, whom I honor deeply for his wisdom, encouragement, and enlightenment through this book and all walks of life. I wish there was some way I could repay all I have received from him, both in spiritual wisdom and friendship. I thank Rita Milios LCSW, for her encouragement and friendship. She is always there when I need her and pushing me along. She is as close to me as a sister. I give special thanks for the woman who helped me tie all this together, Dottie Zimmerman, a true angel and friend. I also give special thanks to Dr. Nancy Kimes; Kwan Yin Reiki Master She will always be a dear life long friend. I want to extend a heart felt thanks to Artist and friend Barb Keener RN, Mary Seibert RN and Richard Demaray- Reiki Master Practitioner, Holly Stuart RN, and E. Flame.

Mostly, I give thanks to each and every nurse in America. Whether you realize it or not, the Nursing profession, at large, is such a wonderful Healing Team. You put forth so much effort into healing of the sick. Allow this book to be a tool towards the Healing Energy that comes back to nourish you as well as your patients.

About the Author

Debbie Glasgow RN, CRMI, CHTP is a Certified Reiki Touch Practitioner - Instructor, Usui Reiki Master teacher, Certified Healing Touch practitioner and cardiac intensive care nurse (for over 10 years). She is the founder of the Reiki Touch For Nurses program, and views it as a bridge between Eastern and Western Medicine. She carries a diploma in Herbal Medicine from the Australian college of Herbal Medicine. Debbie's private practice is located at the International Center for Reiki Touch Training in Ottawa Lake, Michigan. She has taught Reiki throughout the United States and is a member of the Michigan Holistic Nurses Association and the AHNA.

As a young girl she was administering energy touch healing to wounded animals. Her inherent love for animals and healing work may have stemmed from her Cherokee Ancestry. Today she incorporates Reiki Touch healing in her everyday care with her patients and clients. In her private holistic practice, she teaches and practices Reiki Touch, Usui Reiki and other kinds of holistic therapies.

Debbie teaches Reiki Touch for Nurses, a multilevel program for Nurses offering contact hours for each level. Her classes are fun and provide a means for networking with other holistic nurses while learning. Debbie is also one of the founders of ToledoTLC, a nonprofit organization in Ohio dedicated to holistic education for the community. She believes, "Where there is inspiration and desire for positive changes in one's health, the powerful combination of information, caring support, and holistic living can produce incredible results for anyone."

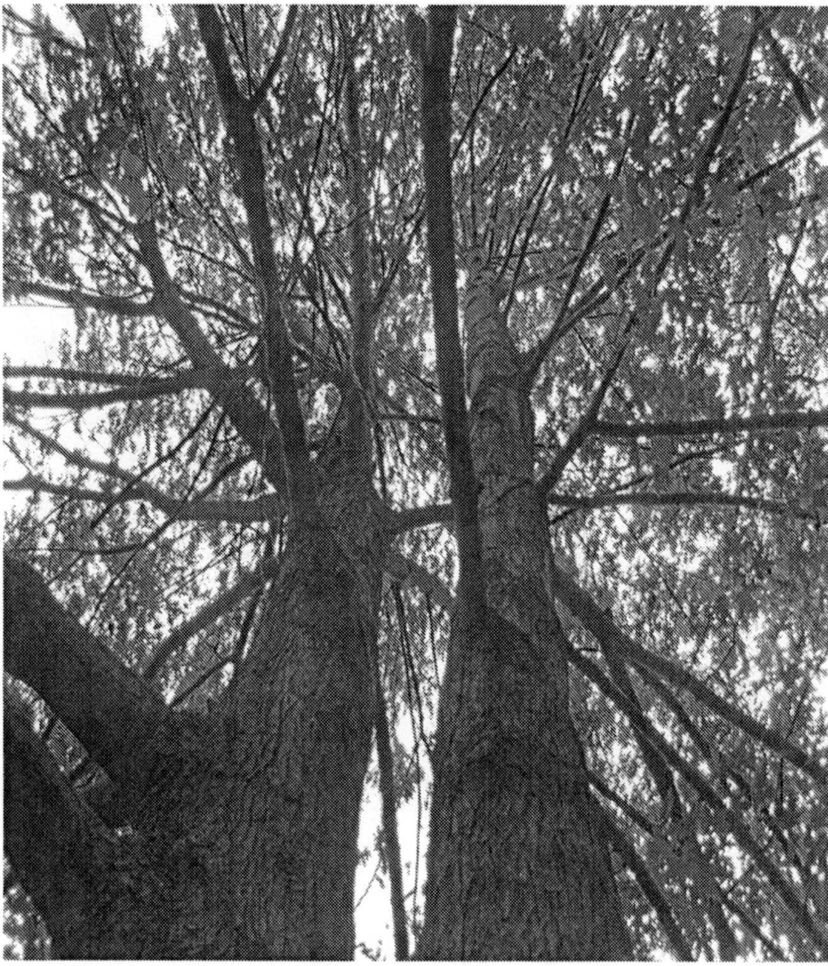

Swaying Tree - by Richelle Reynolds

Fate

Can be

As subtle as the

Swaying of a tree.

Don't try to understand,

Only feel with all your heart

That God is…

Very real…

Very present…

In every moment.

By Richelle Reynolds

Foreword

It is an honor for me to write this forward as Debbie Glasgow RN and founder of Reiki Touch, is one of the most gifted healers I have come to know. When you are in her presence or hear her words you are uplifted as you feel her love and compassion come through like none other. Through the years, Debbie has taught me a great deal on my own journey and has given me many Reiki Touch sessions leaving me in awe of her God-given gift. She has truly integrated her spirit with her humanity.

As a Physician and former patient of a life threatening illness, I know first hand that nurses are the angels of the health care profession, as they work selflessly to care for others. Yet, with the challenges of managed care and the shortage of nurses, the nursing profession has become more challenging. As the front line of the health care system, nurses are constantly feeling the effects of working with the ill, from taking ownership of their patients' problems and stories, to meeting the demands of both their patients and physicians at the same time. Is it no wonder that many nurses are not in optimal health?

I ask you to imagine a picture frame. Into that frame, insert an image of the most important person for whom you need to make important choices. This person can be anyone. There are no exceptions. Who would you choose? If you did not choose yourself, don't you think it's high time that you did? It's time to take care of yourself, while you also bring back high quality, compassionate care for your patients. Through Reiki Touch, Debbie explains how you can do both.

In Reiki Touch, Debbie introduces you to a new way of caring for yourself and for your patients. You will find yourself becoming more at peace, centered and empowered, as you learn to take back your power and become a vessel for healing. This book will introduce you to the Principles of Reiki Touch and you will learn how to allow the energy of nurturing, healing and love, to come through your hands and to your patients. As you give, you receive, and you will be amazed at how your patients respond to Reiki Touch and how recharged you feel at the same time! No longer will you feel drained at the end of the day, but energized as your mind, body and spirit become unified.

Debbie is a true Master teacher and leader in the healing profession. I know you will find the information in this book valuable, just as I have. Reiki Touch was founded and developed for all of you, the nurses, the angels of the health care system. Read this book, take a Reiki Touch workshop from Debbie, and see your own life transform, as well as the lives of your patients.

Namaste',

Dr. Steven Gaynor, DPM, DABPS

Author of "From Physician to Healer"

Founder of "Energetic Diamond Rebalancing"

Reiki Touch Practitioner

Preface

We need to put THE CARE back into health care.

Have you ever thought about what it would be like with the tables turned? What would it feel like if you were the patient? Have you ever tried looking outside the box, rather than just doing your day-to-day mundane duties, as a nurse inside the box? Have you ever thought there might be something to this mind, body, spirit stuff you've been hearing about? There is a wide variety of scientific evidence clearly showing the relationship between physical health, emotions, thought processes and interactions from one human to another.

Years ago I began to see the paradigm of nursing, the need to give compassionate care to the patient verses the hustle, bustle rat race where there is barely enough time to pass medications, help with procedures, yet maintain a high quality of patient care. I realized I wanted to give my patients something more than just routine care. I wanted to be certain they felt their nursing care was professional, safe and compassionate with an added sense of trust. Well the "professional and safe" part is fairly easy and certainly of the utmost importance, yet the compassionate and trusting care can be more of a challenge for many nurses in today's world. Even though patients usually don't voice it, they often feel like they do not get enough personal attention. This may stem from the fast pace of the environment with sophisticated tests and machines and an increased level of technology.

I recall, long ago a patient telling me that he really didn't care if he healed or not because he felt like no one really cared about him anyway. Have you ever thought what that must feel like? Feeling loved, accepted and cared for, plays an important role in a patient's ability to heal. Feelings such as hate, anger, fear and despair all have an affect on the immune system, the energy system, and your entire being. Regardless of your specialty, you should radiate a natural "healing presence" for the patients, others, and yourself. Nurses should nurture the ideas of active listening, empathy, and encouragement to those who are suffering. Using a caring touch can bring all these concepts uniquely together. I offer the wisdom of the principles of "Reiki Touch for Nurses" to be used as a tool for all nurses regardless of background or specialty. You can use this book as an opportunity to understand the relationship between touch and healing. True healing is actually multidimensional. The mind, body, emotions, and spirit all affect you as a whole. By actively bringing these concepts and touch techniques into standard practice, you may be surprised at the healing and heart felt trust that takes place, healing not just the patient, but the nurse as well.

Through this book, I have introduced basic information about the Energy system and how it is used in Reiki Touch Therapy. It is through learning how to fully balance your own energy system that you create the foundation to begin the process of Reiki Touch. The concepts in this book will help you delve deeper into Holistic Nursing. It is through caring for your patient in mind, body, emotion and spirit that the patients' needs are fully meet. As you truly begin to understand and use these skills, you will be able to fully embrace the needs of your patients. Reiki Touch has much to offer the profession of nursing. It can help build a powerful bond between nurse and patient, and to help relax the patient while easing pain, stress and discomfort. Reiki Touch is a way to help enhance the professional care that you already give to your patients. It is used as a complimentary tool to western medicine and in no way takes the place of western medicine. It is rather the bridge that binds eastern and western medicine.

This book also brings into our awareness the importance of the nurse as a role model, addressing attitudes and values that play an integral part of patients perception of their total health care .The intent of this book is to offer a tool which allows nurses to explore another avenue of caring for patients, through communication skills and by enhancing the practice of Nursing with Reiki Touch. It is great pleasure to bring this book into manifestation to further the professional and spiritual growth of nurses, and all who read it.

Chapter 1:

Definition, Benefits and History of Reiki Touch

What is Reiki Touch?

Reiki Touch is an energetic healing modality used to help balance, relax and restore the human energy system. The Japanese word Reiki consist of two kanji: Rei and Ki. Rei means spirit and Ki means energy. The work Reiki then, means spiritual energy.

Reiki Touch is a bridge between Western and Eastern Healing modalities and can easily be used in any health care setting. Reiki Touch is designed for the bedside nurse because it can easily be incorporated with most types of patient care. It can produce powerful effects on all levels of the recipients. These effects contribute to feelings of peacefulness and well being, therefore complimenting Western Medicine.

Nurses use touch to influence the energy system, specifically the energy field that surrounds the body. The non-invasive techniques of Reiki Touch utilize the hands to clear, energize and balance the energy system, therefore affecting physical, mental, emotional and spiritual well being. It is based on a heart-centered relationship in which the patient and nurse come together energetically to facilitate the patient's health. The goal is to restore harmony and balance within the energy system, which allows an alteration in the stress response and pain perception and assist in general healing. These non-invasive techniques aid in transformation towards relaxation and healing.

All living things have life force energy. Reiki Touch helps us to connect with this energy for purpose of mind, body, spirit interaction, and growth. Reiki energy is Spiritual in nature but is not a religion and holds no religious creed or doctrine. Reiki Touch treatments are given with the use of lying on of hands and can actually be used in virtually any clinical setting. This is a natural method providing patients or clients with an opportunity to experience deep relaxation and less pain while quickening the healing process.

Learning and becoming attuned to the Reiki Touch energy through the classes empowers nurses to assist in directing energy, as needed, to the client. This hands on therapy is very non invasive and easy to perform. This therapy has been proven time and time again as an excellent tool for relaxation and pain relief. It also enhances general health and well being, providing the client with a profound sense of peace.

Reiki Touch is noninvasive and very user friendly. It can be administered with the presence of family or other health team members and does not require privacy in order to be administered. It is easy to use and to learn. Reiki Touch is a nursing intervention. The Reiki Touch Program is designed for nurses working in a health care setting. The techniques learned in the more advanced levels may also be used in a private holistic practice.

The Reiki Touch for Nurses program is a multilevel program worth continuing educational hours, providing contact hours for nurses in the United States of America. The classes start with the Introductory level through Master Training level. The more advanced classes bring forth new hybrid information and energy skills that enhance this powerful healing modality. These classes provide contact hours for nurses.

Reiki Touch for nurses COMPLIMENTS conventional health care and is used in collaboration with traditional Western medicine as an adjunctive tool for healing of the mind, emotions, body, and spirit. It does not take the place of Western medicine, rather adds to it in a gentle yet profound way. Reiki Touch is an incredible method of energy healing that joins the nurse and patient at the heart level. The Reiki Touch for Nurses program incorporates much information on the energy system, nervous and endocrine system, as well as touch techniques needed to bring it all together in a scientific, yet holistic manner. Reiki Touch is technically designed for nurses, yet the skills of the hands-on Reiki Touch can actually be taught to anyone with a true intent to assist in the natural healing process.

Note: If you are interested in classes and contact hour information, please check with the Center (see chapter 6 for information)

Benefits of Reiki Touch

This noninvasive therapy can be used regardless of the field of nursing in which you work.

Benefits for the patient:

- Allows for deep relaxation and decreases stress
- Useful by decreasing the amounts for narcotics needed
- Cardiac patients who have just experienced a cardiac event or faced with heart surgery
- Aids in a sense of trust and care between nurse and patient
- Patients with asthma or COPD exacerbation.
- Any and all pre and post surgical patients
- Patients with excruciating pain even though you have medicated them and they are not due for their next dose of medication.
- Oncology patients who suffers with much discomfort and anxiety and needing that additional caring support.
- Useful for rebalancing the energy system after chemotherapy or radiation.
- Patients experiencing headaches including migraines
- Confused elderly patient that you can't medicate due to neurological reasons or a state of delirium
- Delivery room patients experiencing often times uncontrollable pain accompanied by severe anxiety.
- Patients with chronic painful disorders such as fibromyalgia, arthritis, TMJ, etc.
- Newborns or pediatrics who need comfort and reassurance
- Virtually all patients, regardless of diagnosis, can benefit from Reiki Touch

Benefits for the Nurse:

- Nurses deal with personal stress much easier
- Provides the nurse with a sense of balance and healing
- Aids in the Nurses self growth and healing
- Aids in a sense of trust and care between nurse and patient
- Nurses learn more effective communication techniques

Reiki Touch is never harmful, and very easy and acceptable to administer.

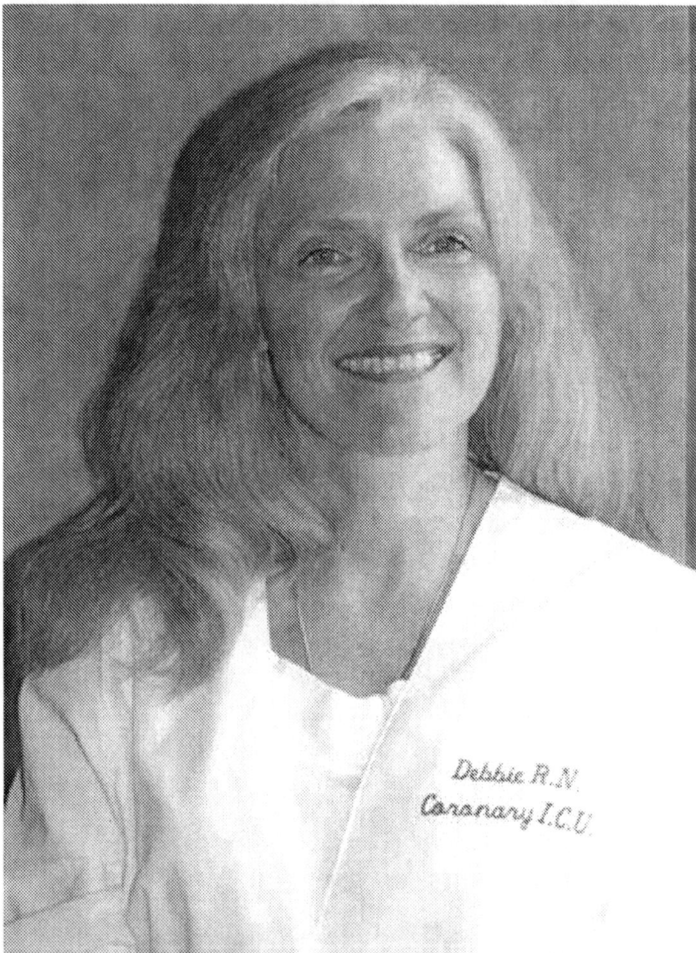

Debbie Glasgow RN, Founder of Reiki Touch for Nurses

ORIGINAL REIKI TOUCH IDEALS

Allow your heart to be filled
With gratitude each day.

Commit yourself to the compassionate
Concern and care for all.

Embrace the healing energy which
Transforms our health, attitudes, values
And beliefs.

Proclaim your healing hands as a
Tool providing peace, healing
And love for all who suffer.

Let only words of kindness come from
Your mouth and energy of compassion and
Love from your heart
To embrace all those
You come in contact with.

Know and trust that you are
A guiding light leading the way towards
Healing, growth, and oneness

~~ **Pray these words from your heart each day** ~~
By Debbie Glasgow, founder of Reiki Touch

Reiki Touch History

Debbie Glasgow RN, Certified Reiki Touch Practitioner and Instructor, Certified Usui Reiki Master, founded The Reiki Touch for Nurses program in December of 2004.For years she utilized a combination of modalities including Healing Touch, Usui Reiki and Therapeutic Touch to aid in stress reduction and overall general healing of the patient. She soon realized the need for simplicity - a type of touch therapy that would be widely accepted in a clinical setting, that would be versatile, effective yet non-invasive This realization gave birth to ~~ what is known today as "Reiki Touch", a simple, yet very effective approach to touch therapy.

Prior to 2004, Debbie worked extensively with Dr. Steven Gaynor, Physician of Podiatry, and Spiritual healer. They worked together on clients in her private practice where they developed techniques that aid in spiritual healing and stress reduction. Some of these techniques were incorporated into the Reiki Touch program, therefore recognizing Dr. Gaynor as very instrumental in the development of this program. In mid September of 2004, during a Healing Reiki share, Debbie received more insight on the techniques to be developed and used in the Reiki Touch for Nurses program. These techniques were received intuitively while performing a deep Reiki treatment on her Reiki Master.

The realization of the great need of healing energy work in the hospitals was greatly recognized by Debbie, Dr. Gaynor and many others.

The original Usui Reiki is a Japanese energetic healing modality, which is widely used throughout the world as a healing touch complimentary therapy. There are many Usui Reiki practitioners both in the medical and non-medical fields. The original Reiki energy probably was discovered in Tibet thousands of years ago. It was then nearly lost over the ages. In the early 1900s Dr Usui, a Buddhist and a Japanese Physician, rediscovered Reiki and termed it Usui Reiki after his name. He earned the title of Grand Master of Usui Reiki. Usui Reiki was then passed from Dr Usui to Dr Hayashi. Hawayo Takata, a student of Dr Hayashi, brought Usui Reiki to America in the mid 1900's.

Debbie Glasgow Received her Usui Reiki Master Certification in 2002. There are just three Reiki Masters between Debbie and Mrs. Takata, so the teachings are extremely close to that of the original teachings of Dr. Usui.

The Reiki Touch for Nurses program includes all the original teachings and content from Usui Reiki, levels one through Master level. It also includes an additional Buddhist and a Hebrew symbol, both channeled in 2004. The new energy of both the Buddhist and Hebrew symbols and their meanings make the Reiki Touch modality so unique.

The Reiki Touch for Nurses is different from Usui Reiki and Healing Touch in a sense that some of the delivery fashion is different, in order to meet the needs of the patient in the health care clinical environment. Reiki Touch is increasingly recognized as one of the most widely researched and applied techniques for stress reduction, pain reduction and healing. Nurses have traditionally been at the forefront in patient care and *Reiki Touch* emphasizes the value of this elegant, simple approach to energy healing work.

The Reiki Touch for Nurses program also includes detailed information of the human energy system and valuable information on concepts that help increase communication, trust and a positive attitude between Nurses, patients, and other members of the health care team.

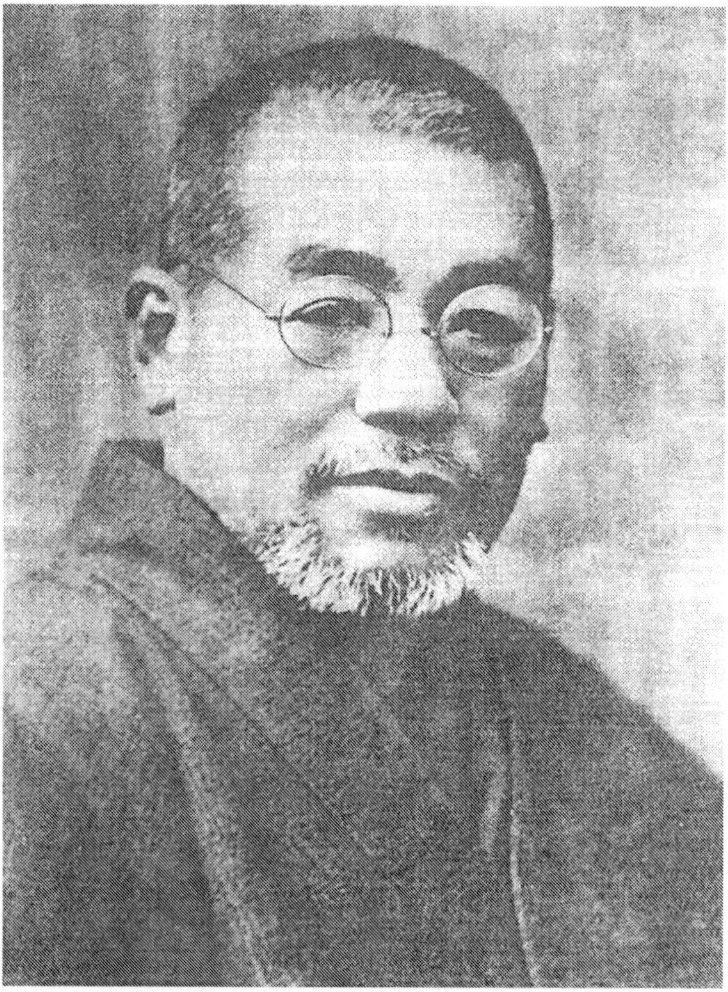

Mikao Usui: Founder of Usui Reiki

The Original Usui Reiki Ideals …quote by Dr Usui:

The secret method of inviting in happiness and the wonderful medicine for all diseases of body, mind and soul

Just for today, do not be angry.

Do not worry and be filled with gratitude.

Devote yourself to your work

And be kind to others.

Every morning and every evening

Join your hands in prayer,

Pray these words to your heart,

And chant these words with your mouth.

Dr. Usui wrote these five Reiki principles

He clearly brings out the five principles as

JUST FOR TODAY

1) Don't get angry
2) Don't worry
3) Show appreciation
4) Work hard (including on yourself)
5) Be kind to others

He taught that one should sit in the gassho position mornings and evenings and repeat these words out loud and in your heart

Dr Usui believed this affirmation, the original Usui Reiki ideas, to be a key factor in improving body and mind. He also believed and taught the importance of balance, harmony and preventive therapy in the maintenance of total health of the holistic you. "Holistic you" refers to mind, body, spirit and emotion. When one of these is out of balance, it inadvertently has an affect on the other parts of the "Holistic you".

Little is known about the life of Dr. Usui, however the facts we do know came from much research in Japan. We know he was born August 15th, 1865 in the Japanese province in Gifu. On March 9, 1926 he died in Fukuyama as a result of a cerebral accident. He began teaching Reiki around the year 1920 after receiving the Reiki information during a very long meditation and fasting period. In 1921, he opened a Reiki practice in Harajuku, Tokyo, close to Meiji Jingu (Meiji shrine).

He believed that in all situations in life, it is wise to allow ourselves to be guided by our hearts and not our ego. In the heart as the spiritual center of the human being, there is no place for duality; there are no money or power struggles, no anger, hatred or greed or other ego based feelings. He found the inner wisdom and understanding that can only be achieved when a person follows his own light, heart and trusts in his own journey. He lived a truly spiritual life and understood that wisdom and true knowledge can only be comprehended when the body, mind, and heart are in harmony and unity with each other. He was dedicated to being open and receptive and living in the present moment. Dr Usui believed when we are in disharmony in body, mind or spirit, there is a cascade of events that take place that causes energetic blocks in the energy system and eventually the physical body.

He taught that if we keep our thoughts pure and healthy and lived a balanced, wholesome, loving life, that health and well-being would prevail. All would be in harmony and homeostasis, including the physical body. Through harmony and balance of the energy system we maintain health, well-being and happiness.

Today, Reiki Touch is viewed as a bridge between Eastern and Western practices.

Chapter 2:

The Human Energy System

Intangible, Invisible, Infinite, Ignition of life. …

It sustains each of us …all the time

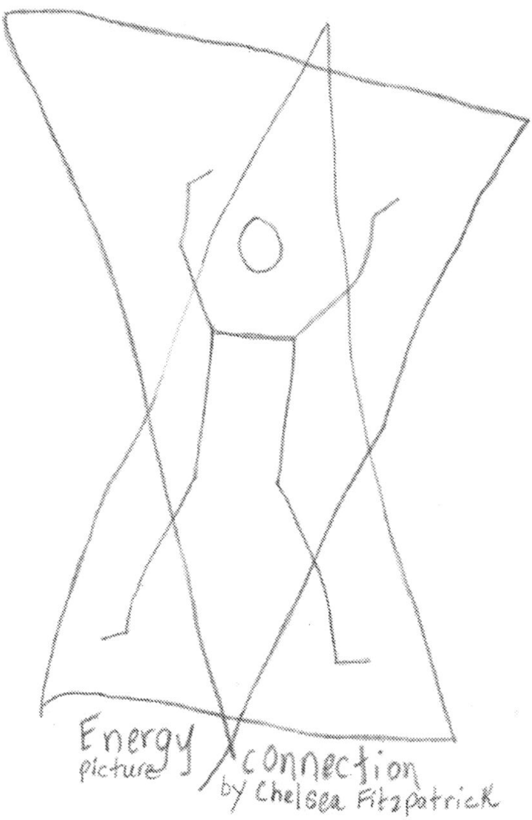

Figure 1: Energy Connection by Chelsea Fitzpatrick

You might be asking yourself, why is it important for me to know about the Human energy system? You, the nurse, have a great ability to work with patients on an energetic level because you have a great deal of contact with them. As a health care provider, you can address the patient as a holistic being, not just a physical being.

The Human Energy system is just as important as the other systems of the human body. It works with all the other systems all the time. They are all interconnected. The respiratory, circulatory, endocrine, eliminatory, skeletal, nervous, digestive and energy systems **all work together** to maintain homeostasis in our beings. The "energy system" is the "invisible system," because we cannot see it with our naked eye. However, it can be viewed by Kerlian photography, which we will discuss later. We are holistic beings of body, mind, emotions and spirit. With all of our sophisticated technology, we can easily visualize any and all parts of the physical body; hair, skin, eyes, organs, tissues, cells, essentially every physical component. For most however, we cannot visualize the other very important counterparts – the emotions, the mind and the spirit. Just because we cannot see the energy system does not mean it does not exist. We all have a MENTAL body, (or mental auric field) an EMOTIONAL body (or an emotional auric field), a SPIRITUAL body (or called a spiritual auric field). The terms body or auric fields are interchangeable. All of the systems have an "energetic and automatic" affect on the other systems. We are interconnected, intricate, holistic beings. We cannot separate these. It would be like trying to separate your aorta from your heart. One system depends on the other. Much like a car depends on the engine, tires and steering wheel to function, the human body depends on **ALL** of its systems to function at its highest capacity to maintain homeostasis and health, at all time.

Energetically, there are two worlds, the INNER world and the OUTER world. Most of us are constantly living in reaction to what happens in our **outer** world. We falsely believe that our outer world will determine how we feel; whether we will be sad, happy, pleased or fearful. The list goes on and on. Happiness, confidence and fear do not exist in the **outer** world. We cannot purchase or touch them. We can only experience these feelings in our **inner** world ~ our emotions, our consciousness. Our inner world is the combination of our thoughts, feelings, perceptions, attitudes and beliefs ~ OUR CONSCIOUSNESS. True balance and power begin when we can control our inner world, when we can control the way we act, react, think and feel, regardless of what happens outside of us. Yes, the outer world does affect our inner world, but our inner world also affects our outer world, what we experience and create in our life. When we master and control our inner world, we shape our own outer world. It is not what happens to you that determines your happiness; rather the way you **respond** to what happens in your environment you that determines this. With awareness, intent provides the root in which your journey will unfold and manifest. Thoughts are things and the seat of power resides in your thoughts. In a sense, we create and manifest our outer worlds all the time, every moment. If we think and focus on a positive attitude with healthy thoughts, there is more of a likelihood this is what will manifest. On the other hand, if we think negative thoughts and harvest ideas of poor health, despair, sadness or fear, it is likely to also to manifest. It is simple, thoughts are energy.

Energetically, we are the masters of our own creation; our own happiness, our own sadness. We choose to love or hate. We choose to embrace or reject. We choose to stay or go. It's all about choices.

We are all intricate beings of multilevel consciousness. We all possess and come into this lifetime with "universal life force" also called " life force energy". This life force energy is the sustenance of the Energy System, much like blood is the sustenance of the circulatory system. Life force is the vital energy contained in all living things and circulates through the energy system. This invisible system helps keep you alive. The energy system is a highly complex system, which acts as the ignition for all other physical systems of the human body. It is the energy system, which allows the physical body access to universal life force energy. This universal life energy is found everywhere and sustains all forms of life. It is in, on and around you. This "invisible" system consists of Chakras, Bioenergy fields (also called auras), Meridians and Nadias. These four parts of the energy system work with a vital force called UNIVERSAL ENERGY (or called universal life energy), which is vital for sustaining life and useful for maintaining health and overall balance and homeostasis. By understanding and working with our energy systems, we can help our bodies maintain balance and fertilize its own homeostatic mechanisms, which eventually aid in the entire healing process.

What is Energy?

Lets discuss ENERGY before we get into the intricate parts of the Energy system. I am often asked, "What is energy?" It's somewhat a difficult concept, much like trying to describe love. At any rate it is the force that binds all creation. It is the life force that dwells within and without all living things. All living things, without exceptions share in a generalized Life-Energy Field, in the same way that all physical objects in space are subject to gravity. This life energy flows naturally around us and through our energy systems. It is the life force that exists within each and every molecule. It cannot be created or destroyed and is in a constant state of change. If you look at Einstein's work it is clear that mass is energy. Energy can change shape and form yet not be destroyed and it exists everywhere. Everything is energy. Everything in the universe is made up of atoms. Inside of each atom are electromagnetic charges – protons, electrons and neutrons. Groups of atoms form molecules. Therefore, everything is energy and is in constant vibration. Your pencil, paper, clothes, food, and your human body are all vibrations of energy. Everything can be measured as vibrational energy ~~ as a frequency. Quantum physics has revealed that everything-ALL forms of life and objects, from the solid mass of the earth to every object and being on it- pulses with energetic frequencies. You, the people and places around you, even this book – all resonate with energy. And that energy moves outward from you, in space and time, attracting and responding to the other energies in the cosmos.

So someone who is happy will be vibrating in a different level of energy or frequency than someone who is depressed, angry or fearful. Our energies are constantly interacting and impacting each other. For an example, if you are with a group of friends laughing and having a good time, and suddenly a person comes in with a nasty or angry attitude, soon the energy or "mood" of the group changes. The energy may become negative or of a lower vibration. Many times this type of energy can be felt, even without words. Our thoughts and emotions hold an energetic vibration. Like tends to attract like. To give another example, have you ever been in a sad or low vibrational mood and just the right person or music has come along and you felt your mood change? We also know people who are definitely NOT fun to be around. There is heaviness to their presence, an agitation to their energy. They often have us feeling dissatisfied and drained, as if something has been taken away, instead of given to us. These are the energy vampires. They send out hateful signals because, no matter how they behave, they inwardly are hateful to themselves. All of this is the inescapable *law of magnetism*. In your career, health, financial status, home and relationships, what you find yourself experiencing, will always be an outward manifestation of the energy that you, yourself are creating on a daily basis.

According to Taber's Cyclopedic Medical Dictionary, Energy is described like this:

'Energy- The capacity of a system for doing work. Energy exists in various forms such as kinetic, potential, light, heat, ionized radiation, and sound. Changes in energy may manifest physically, chemically or both. Conservation of energy further explains that energy cannot be created or destroyed, but is transformed into other forms. Kinetic energy is the energy of motion. Latent energy is energy that exists yet is not being used.

Potential energy is stored energy. Radiant energy is energy transmitted through space. Some examples of this are radio waves, infrared waves, gamma rays and cosmic rays.'

In this same medical dictionary I also found the definition of Energy Field Disturbance:

Energy Field Disturbance- a putative disruption of the flow of energy surrounding a persons being that results in a disharmony of the body, mind, and or spirit.

This dictionary then refers you to the back of the book into "The Nursing diagnosis of Energy Field Disturbance" which gives the following information~

~~~~ *Diagnostic Division~Ego, Integrity*

'Definition: A disruption of the flow of energy (Aura) surrounding a persons being that results in a disharmony of the body, mind and or spirit.

RELATED FACTORS Blocks in energy fields, Depression, Increased state of anxiety, impaired immune system and or pain.'

DEFINING CHARACTERISTICS OF ENERGY FIELD DISTURBANCES:

'Objective ~ Temperature change, (warmth or coolness), Visual change, (image, color): disruption of the field (vacant, hole, spike, bulge): Movement (wave/spike/tingling/dense/flowing): Sounds (tones, words)'
~~~~

Now if the medical dictionaries are recognizing the importance of including the Energy system and how it is used in a nursing diagnosis, it must hold value. Now, the next time someone says to me, " I don't know if I believe in energy fields or auras" Let me just refer them to pages 2611 and 681 in Tabers Edition 19. The energy system is acknowledged as fact in many prominent medical publications including college textbooks, science, and medical and Nursing journals. This book is written in an objective rather than subjective manner. Multiple successful Bioenergy findings have been confirmed at many major universities, including The Medical Sciences Academy in Moscow, and are supported by research in Great Britain, Netherlands, Germany, Poland, Russia, and the United States.

In Eastern culture, energy is explained as Universal life energy that sustains all living organisms. Although, the idea of subtle vital energy is only just now being accepted and used in western medicine, it has long been a feature of eastern systems. In India for example the energy is called Prana or Ki. Other countries refer to it as chi or Qi (pronounced Chi). So, to further clarify, Ki, Qi, Chi (all pronounced as Chi) prana, life force, and universal energy are all interchangeable. There is even yet another more condensed form of stored chi energy that sits at the base of the spine called Kundalini energy. People that practice Yoga are familiar with this stored energy. One popular form of Yoga that works specifically with the release of this stored Chi energy is Kundalini Yoga.

We are constantly, every moment, attempting to balance our energy system. This takes place either on a conscious or unconscious level. For example, if one feels emotional pain or despair, tears may manifest. The tears act as a release button that allows the emotion to flow. All systems in the body, including the energy system are endlessly trying to maintain homeostasis. (or balance towards health maintenance).

"Reiki Touch" is an energetic healing modality used to help balance and restore the human energy system. After reading about energy you still may be out in left field, I don't blame you because I was too, at first. It is much easier to understand chess once you have played it a few times, much like working with the energy system. Give yourself a chance to learn about it, and then apply it. Feel what it feels like and review the results, then decide for yourself weather it can be of benefit for you and or your patient or both. Now that we have an idea of what energy is, lets talk about the different *parts* of the Energy system.

The Energy System consists of four basic subgroups, which we will discuss one at a time. The bioenergy fields (also called energy fields, human energy fields, aura, auric fields or energy layers) chakras, nadias, and meridians are all very important parts of the energy system. All of these subgroups (parts) work very closely together. Each part of the system has it's own subjective role and function, yet are still an integral part of each other. The Energy system works with all the other systems, primarily the Endocrine system.

The Bioenergy Fields (Aura)

We, as humans are enveloped in an energetic sheath known as the "aura". This aura or sheath is similar to the atmosphere, which surrounds and protects the earth. There are layers of energy within the atmosphere, which sustain and nourish life on this planet. It would be impossible for life to exist on this planet without these layers of energy. Like the earth, we as humans are also enveloped in layers or fields of energy, which protects us and gives us boundaries and existence. The human bioenergy fields or "aura" plays an integral part of the functioning of the Energy system.

When you feel loved, charismatic, and happy, your aura could easily fill the room. When you feel up, energetic and on top of things, your aura is big, wide, healthy, and vibrant. Likewise, when you are sad, depressed or down, your aura is down also. It will become smaller, closer to your physical being. It may only extend out a couple feet whereas usually your energy fields may extend out much further (say 5 or 6 feet depending on your own personal aura). Your aura automatically acts to embrace and protect you.

With some practice, you can begin to feel the energy field around yourself and others. Picture it as a shell around your body and visualize it getting bigger and moving away from you. Use deep breathing as you perform this. As you exhale, see the shell moving away from your physical being. Try this sometime.

Your Bioenergy fields, (also called Human Energy Fields-HEF), are multi-layered spheres of energy that emanate from your physical body and interact with the atmosphere around you. It is very protective and embraces you, filtering out certain energies and also drawing in other energies at the same time. The Chakras on the other hand are "energy centers" which are attuned to much higher vibrations. The aura acts like a two-way antenna because it brings energy from the environment into your chakras, and also sends energy from the chakras outwardly into the environment and other energy fields.

Many experts have scientifically investigated the human aura. One expert, Valerie Hunt, a neurophysiologist conducted meticulous studies at UCLA's Energy Fields Laboratory, over a twenty year period. Her studies compared aura readings with neuropsychological measures. The colors seen by the clairvoyant experts matched *exactly* with electromyography (EMG) wave patterns picked up by the electrodes on the skin at the spots being observed. (Valerie Hunt, Infinite Mind, 1995). Psychologist Dorothy Gundling, in 1977, found that experts saw changes in size, color and shape of the energy fields in relationship due to stress or happy feelings. There were consistent reports of SHIFTS OR CHANGES IN THE AURA. For example, when a person is under stress, or experiences changes in their environment, or when a person has energy healing work done on them, there will be changes that occur in the auric fields. These observations also corresponded with blood pressure, pulse rate, respiratory rate, and brain wave patterns. She also found that music and meditation produced changes in the energy fields. The combined use of biofeedback sensors, Kerlian photography and other special computing equipment has clearly demonstrated shifts and changes in color, shapes and size of the energy fields after the application of hands on energy work, prayer, and or acupressure. The HEF changes and shifts with changes in thought patterns, moods, and environmental factors. Your auric field may change when you are in close proximity with another individual because their energy fields combine or overlap with your energy fields. Have you ever noticed your own mood change when you are in the presence of certain people? Your energy fields constantly blend with the energy fields of those you encounter.

The HEF are intrinsic layers, which we could discuss at great length yet I will only briefly discuss them due to the nature of this book. Keep in mind; the words layers, fields, or aura or energy fields are sometimes used interchangeably. Energy fields surround each and every one of us. Most people cannot see them, but they are there. Some of us can feel them and that is the basis for the Reiki Touch work. You learn as a practitioner to " feel or sense the field ". One of the capabilities of the energy fields is to transport energies from around our body into another persons energy system, or into the environment. The energy fields can also be used as a means to transport energy from the universe into our energy fields and physical body. These fields also have the capability to store energy, release energy and provide a protective mechanism of the physical body (Donna Eden, 1998).

The first four layers of the human energy fields are the Etheric (also called Vital or Subtle layer), Emotional layer (or Emotional field) the Mental layer, and the Astral layer (also called Intuitive or Spiritual layer). The astral layer connects energetically with the heart chakra. This layer is the bridge layer, which allows a blending of energies into the spiritual plane and the physical plane. The fields (or layers), which vibrate with the physical plane, are the vital, emotional and mental fields. If you notice, there are three fields beneath the astral layer and three fields outside of it. The layers outside of the astral are all of very spiritual nature. The layer closest to, and just outside of the astral, is the fifth layer, the Etheric template. It is the physical aspect of the last three layers. The sixth layer is the Celestial layer, which is also the emotional aspect of the higher spiritual layers. The seventh layer is the Ketheric body, which is the mental aspect of the higher spiritual layers. Energy (chi) flows back and forth from the chakras through the layers of the energy fields and vise versa to create balance throughout he energy system and homeostasis for our entire being. Each auric layer has it's own function and is associated with a major chakra. Each chakra is associated with an endocrine gland. There are seven major energy fields and seven major chakras, each corresponding with each other. Illness can result from blocked, weakened, stagnant, or imbalanced energy flow. There are many factors that can influence our energy fields. These are called " factors within and factors without", (which we will discuss in the next chapter). Imbalanced energy flow affects not only the energy system, but other systems as well, which can eventually lead to health breakdown.

The Subtle layer (also called Vital layer or Etheric field) is the first layer, and closest to our physical body. This field interfaces with the emotional field. This vital (or subtle) field extends about 2 to 3 inches from the skin and is the field most often associated with energy balancing or healing work. It has been viewed from different shades of blue to gray. Its shape is the exact same shape as our physical body.

Its main purpose is to act as a protective shield against potentially harmful energy (much like the ozone and the earth) and it easily transports energies in and out from the chakras to the other energy fields and the environment and vice-versa Any deficiencies or blocked energy flow in this layer can have a great impact on proper energy flow into and or out of the chakra, therefore impeding energy flow into the endocrine system and the glands. As a result, illness can result from blocked, weakened, stagnant, or imbalanced energy flow. The subtle layer mostly corresponds with the first chakra, which is the root chakra of the energy system. This layer also corresponds and protects all chakras and the physical body itself. It is the last final protective shield we have against any energies, which may be in the surrounding area, which are not for our highest good. This layer may become very traumatized especially in the case of an amputation. Even though the body part is removed, the aura stays the same, causing confliction within the energy system. Phantom pain is a type of pain one feels even after an extremity has been removed for years. Many are still studying the correlation between this pain and the subtle energy field.

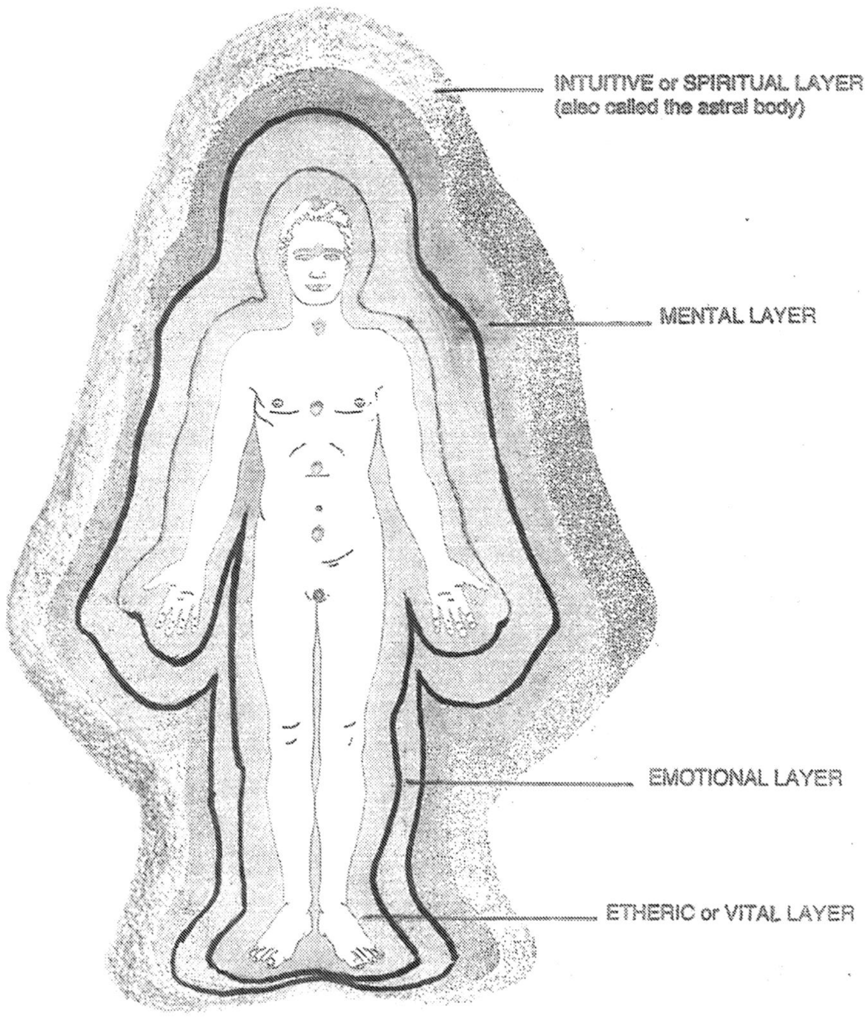

The Four Major Layers of the Human Energy Field

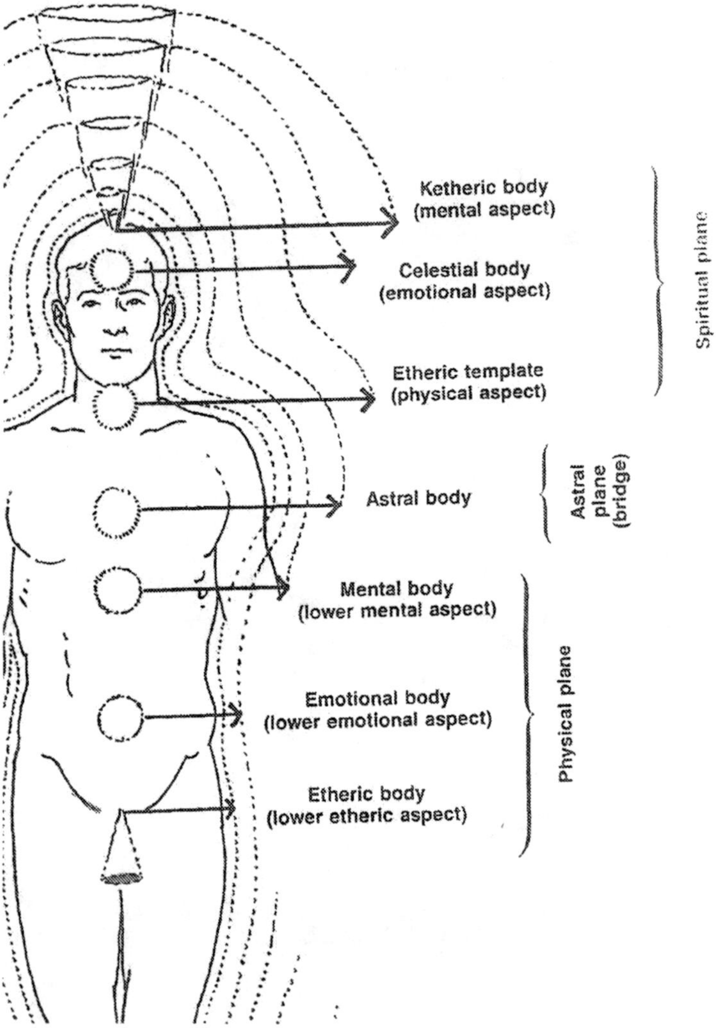

The Seven Layer Auric System (diagnostic view)

The Emotional layer, which extends out from the vital layer has been viewed as a rainbow of colors. This second field (layer) interfaces with the vital (also called subtle or etheric) and the mental layer and at times they overlap as in any of the fields that are next to each other. This field holds the individual's emotional feelings, and general affect. The Emotional layer (field) corresponds to the sacral chakra of the energy system. The thickness or size of it varies from one individual to another. It is often noted to be about 3 to 6 inches away from the physical body. The size and shape of it also changes depending upon your own personal vibration and / or mood at the time. Remember the tone, size and the feel of it changes almost constantly in relationship to our changing feelings and surroundings. If you want another individual to feel what you are feeling, stand or sit in this area. This person will more likely feel your emotion and energetic vibration. Much of the stagnant or blocked energy in this field, including the sacral chakra, is frequently related to emotional stress. This field is cleared and balanced frequently during Reiki Touch energy work.

The Mental layer, which extends out from the emotional layer, lies between the emotional and astral layer. Experts have viewed it as a yellowish color. This third layer embodies our thinking patterns and visual imagery. Like the emotional layer, the size and depth of it may vary depending on the person. This field stands out about 6 to 18 inches away from the physical body. Note that the distance or thickness of each field varies from person to person, and this field is affected by our mental state or disposition at the time. There can be a wide variance in the thickness of this field. An experienced energy practitioner will become very proficient at "feeling" where one field stops and the next begins. If you really want to get your thoughts

across to an individual, talk to him or her while standing in this mental field. Actually for most of us, this comes naturally without even thinking about it. We seem to naturally migrate into this field when exchanging thoughts with another.
This layer corresponds with the solar plexus chakra of the energy system. If you find your thoughts becoming more emotionally based, you will probably find yourself stepping into the other persons vibration……. a little closer, naturally.

The Astral layer (also called the astral body, intuitive layer, or spiritual layer) is the fourth layer that correlates with the heart. This layer extends about 18 to 24 inches away from the physical body. Experts have viewed it as a beautiful cobalt blue in color. This layer holds the energy of love and corresponds to the Heart chakra. It is the layer that is actually the bridge between the physical auric layers and the higher spiritual dimensions.

The last three layers are highly spiritual layers. They are the Etheric Template (5th level), extends out about 22 to 28 inches, the Celestial body (6th layer) which extends out about 28 to 36 inches, and the Ketheric Template or also called the Casual body, which extends out about 3 to 4 feet from the physical body. The energy fields - 5 through 7 are connected with the last 3 chakras, crown, brow, and throat, respectively and are in alignment with the higher spiritual realms. They are associated with free will and energies of a much higher vibration.

The Astral field connects with the heart chakra and is a connecting point between the spiritual fields and the lower physical fields

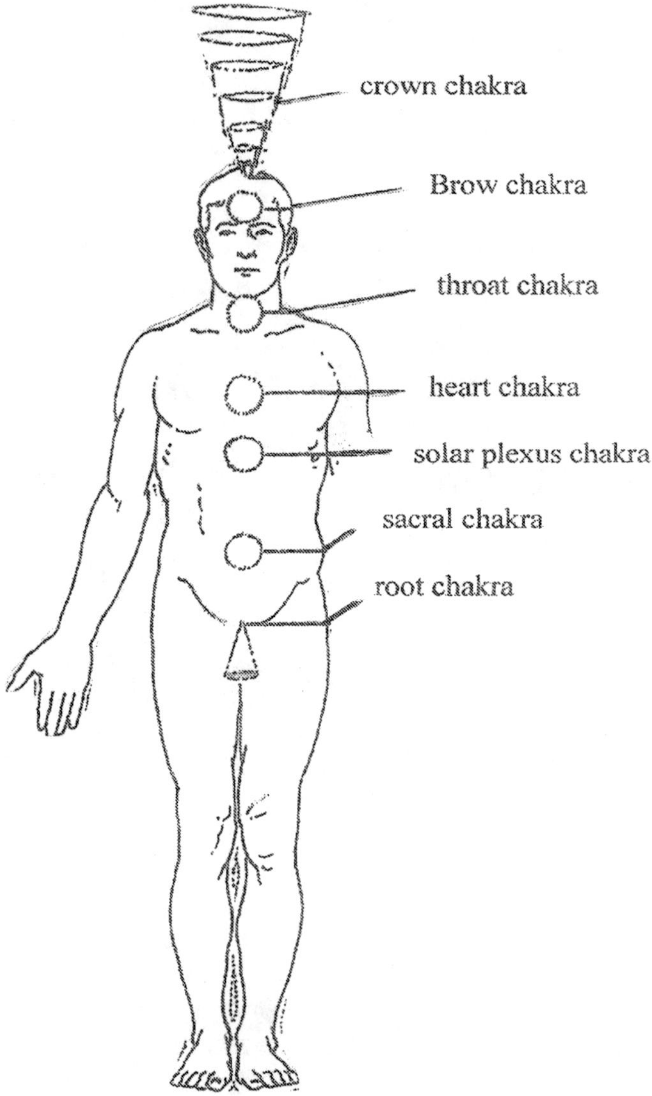
crown chakra
Brow chakra
throat chakra
heart chakra
solar plexus chakra
sacral chakra
root chakra

Chakras

The Chakras

Spinning Round and Round, Transforming, Stimulating, Allowing in Vibrancy and Change

The word Chakra is a Sanskrit word which means wheel, vortex or disk. These wheels allow energy to spin in a certain direction. CHAKRAS ARE CONSENTRATED ENERGY CENTERS. The human body includes hundreds of these energy centers. The major seven chakras in the human body are located from the base of the spine to the top of the head, within our central channel. The chakras RECEIVE, TRANSMIT AND PROCESS energy. Our HEF (human energy fields) and our chakras work very closely with one another to attempt to maintain balance with each other and with the physical body. The Etheric (vital) body is the atmospheric body just outside of the physical body and works with all our chakras. The chakras are connected to specific areas of our consciousness. All the chakras work with each other yet still have their own distinctive function and characteristics. Each chakra is related to at least one gland or more, which then further energizes and nourishes our organs. All the chakras relate to at least one or more of the color spectrum. The chakras allow emotional, mental, spiritual, and physical energy to flow into and out of our physical bodies. Our belief system and attitudes play a role in this function because our beliefs and attitudes hold emotional, mental or spiritual energy. These energies have an impact on our organs, tissues, and cells. The chakras open into the areas of our consciousness as well as areas of our sub-consciousness. This is why prayer, affirmations, meditation, thoughts and spoken words are all vital to our balance and health.

Knowledge of the chakras dates back thousands of years ago. Western culture has inherited the chakra information from Eastern medicine and Yoga disciplines. The chakras are an essential part of the bioenergy system. When you understand how chakras relate to energy and homeostasis, you are then able to utilize chi energy for the benefit of health, balance, and well-being. The main focus here will be on the major chakras. Colors, as a component of the chakras, can be used to soothe, stimulate, and balance each chakra.

We as health care providers are beginning to see the validation of the energy system and the chakras due to modern technology and our changing evolution. Not so long ago the chakras were looked at as mystical and esoteric. We are now becoming more aware of the true mind, body spirit connection. Knowledge of the Energy system and chakras helps bring all of this into perspective. Remember the Energy system works with the other physical systems to maintain health and homeostasis. One system is not more important than the other. They are all essential to health maintenance and sustaining life.

Chakras are vortexes of energy that normally spin like a wheel of energy, clockwise. The seven major ones from the coccyx up are: root chakra (also called base chakra), sacral (navel or womb chakra), solar plexus, heart chakra, throat chakra, brow (third eye) chakra, and crown chakra. Each chakra is associated with a major nerve plexus and endocrine gland and each one also correlates with at least one specific color. Each chakra functions to perform it's own special kind of work with specific types of energy. At the same time, however, all of the charkas help each other as needed. I think of it like making donuts, the baker bakes the shell and the decorator fills them with jelly and the waitress delivers them allowing the customer to eat them. They all function at specific levels and are also able to communicate and help each other as needed. (Unless of coarse the baker calls in sick and the decorator gets stuck baking and filling the donuts).

The function of the chakras is to receive, gather, process, transmit and release energy acting like transformers. The chakras feed the life force energy into and out of the endocrine system, which in turn stimulates or regulates hormonal balance, and maintains homeostasis and health. Each of the chakras are conduits for a particular type of universal energy. The seven major charkas respectively resonate with the principles of survival, (base or root), creativity (sacral), power (solar plexus), love (heart), self expression (throat), transcendence (third eye) and unity (crown). The chakras are specific subtle energy channels which allow energies to flow through them, (if they are working properly), and into the cellular structure of the physical body. The chakras function as energy transformers because they help transform energy from one form and frequency to a higher or lower form and frequency. This energy eventually travels through the endocrine system where it is further transformed into physiological and ultimately cellular changes through the tissues and body. There are virtually hundreds of chakras through out the body. It is important at this point to understand that when the energy system is balanced and free flowing, **ENDORPHINES** are released into the blood . Endorphins act as a foundation in which to gain a stress free environment, provide comfort and assist in the strength of the immune system. An endorphin is a polypeptide produced in the brain that acts as an opiate and produces analgesia by binding to opiate receptor sites involved in pain perception. The threshold for pain is therefore increased by this action. The most active of these compounds is beta-endorphins.

All chakras, when functioning at their highest capacity usually spin clockwise. When they become blocked, as in ill health or disease however, they may spin backwards or much smaller than normal and in the worst-case scenario, not at all. It is through proper assessment of the chakras and energy fields that the practitioner is able to fine-tune the needed work at hand and assist in the release of blockages or stagnant energy. The practitioner's ability to perform a skillful energy assessment takes much practice and persistence. As the client releases stagnant or blocked energy, this allows for balance and free flowing energy within the energy system, therefore assisting with homeostasis.

We are connected in Mind, Body, Spirit and Emotion

All are an integral part of our Total Health

The Root (Base) Chakra

The security center

Being connected and rooted in life

The root chakra is located at the base of the spine in the perineum. It has a funnel shape, which is directed towards the earth. The color red correlates with this energy center. This chakra is connected to the subtle (vital) energy field, and resonates with the element of earth. In the yogic tradition, this chakra is called the *Maladhara*, which means the manifestation of life and energy and the survival instinct. The root provides support for the proper foundation for the journey upward. This chakra energizes and nourishes the adrenal glands for the most part and also provides some energy to the gonads. The gonads are the ovaries and testes, which are the glands of reproduction. The root chakra also helps to provide energy into the lower parts of our bodies –the feet, legs, and hips.

This Energy center corresponds energetically to our sense of belonging to the earth, the will to survive; the fight or flight response in relationship to the hormones released from the adrenal glands. This energy center resonates with feelings of security, wanting to be here and alive, structure, and order, consistency, patience, commitment, stability and manifestation. The root chakra, when healthy and balanced, will allow you to feel connected to this world, happiness, gratitude, and a joy for life.

When this chakra is imbalanced or blocked energetically one may experience low back discomfort, leg or foot pain, depression, family, job or home insecurities. It is surprising the correlation is sometimes seen in people that "have no will to live" will have an imbalance in this particular chakra. The following is an affirmation one can use to energize and balance the root chakra.

Imagine the root chakra spinning clockwise, like a red cone, at the base of your spine as you practice the following affirmation. All affirmations may be said out loud or silently.

"I love myself"

"I am safe and secure at all times"

"I feel grounded in my own power"

"Life is good"

"I feel secure and powerful on all levels of physical, financial, mental and emotional levels."

"I have a strong foundation in this life"

"I love myself"

The Sacral Chakra

Yin / Yang balancing center

I am you and you are me, together we are we

This chakra is located in the sacral region, below the umbilicus and above the root chakra and it resonates with the element of water, which holds emotional passion. This chakra vibrates with the color orange and is connected to the life force of the emotional layer of the energy fields. In the yogic tradition it is called *svadhisthana,* which means finding oneness among duality. This energy center helps is balance our different female and male energies and it corresponds energetically to our sexuality and relationships with others. It helps us to be discerning between helpful and unhelpful influences in our lives. This center helps us in choosing our friends, partners, and acquaintances on an energetic level. It also corresponds with feelings of prosperity, pleasure, and well-being. The sacral chakra works energetically with the kidneys, bladder, and the large intestines. The gonads, which are the endocrine glands of sexuality and reproduction, are energized and nourished by the sacral chakra. It also helps with the functions of balance, assimilation of fluids and nutrients in the large intestines.

The following affirmation is helpful in keeping the sacral chakra balanced and healthy. Try visualizing this chakra glowing with an orange color and spinning clockwise while using the following affirmation:

"I love myself"

"I am willing to allow pleasure and fun into my life"

"Who I am, is enough"

"Life is abundant"

"I am filled with joy and prosperity"

"I attract positive people and situations in my life"

" I feel balanced in my life"

"I love myself"

The Solar Plexus Chakra

The Power Center

The solar plexus is the third chakra and is located in the abdominal region, just under the sternum. This chakra resonates with the element - fire. The yogic name associated with it is *manipura*, which means burning through the resistance of duality and finding ones own strength and transcending the ego. It corresponds with the color yellow. The pancreas is the gland that is energized and nourished by the solar plexus chakra. This chakra holds the energy of discrimination and assertion, which is why it is referred to as the power chakra. It is in this chakra that the tensions about " who I am" and "who others expect me to be" are continually at struggle. This chakra also energizes and nourishes the spleen, liver, gallbladder, and stomach, assisting in digestion and glucose distribution. This center energetically corresponds to our sense of ego, power, courage, identity, fears, and strengths. It is connected to and works closely with the mental layer of our energy field. The third chakra is logical rather than emotional or artistic. It aids in mental clarity and functioning

The following is an affirmation, which can be used to balance and energize the solar plexus. Visualize the color yellow in this charka, spinning clockwise, like a vortex, while you say the following affirmation.

"I love myself"

"I am willing to allow pleasure and fun into my life"

"Who I am, is enough"

"Life is abundant"

"I am filled with joy and prosperity"

"I attract positive people and situations in my life"

"I love myself"

The Heart Chakra
The love center

Energy that flows like the River

In the yogic tradition this chakra is also called the *anahata,* which means unstruck or unhurt, compassionate, soft tender and deep. This chakra resonates with the element – air. It is associated with the color green or pink. It is located between the nipples, in the center of the chest wall. Energetically it is connected to the 4th energy field, which is the astral field, which holds the energy of love and is the bridge between the physical dimensions and the higher more spiritual planes of existence. It corresponds with the thymus gland, an endocrine gland, which also stimulates the immune system. This chakra is associated with the proper functioning of the cardiovascular, respiratory and the immune system. The heart represents unconditional love, forgiveness, devotion, universal love, purity, innocence, harmony, and brotherhood.

When this chakra is blocked or unbalanced, there may be physical manifestations of heart, immunity, or respiratory problems. People who are hostile, angry or fearful often times will have imbalances in this chakra.

Visualize the color green or pink in this chakra as you mentally spin this energy clockwise say the following affirmation for the heart chakra. This is especially helpful with those wanting to create a balance of love and harmony in their lives.

"I love myself"

"Love is purposeful in my life"

"I am open to receiving love"

"I freely give love"

"I give and receive love without judgment"

"I feel at ease with giving and receiving love"

"I love myself"

Throat Chakra
The expression center

Perfect ~~ self expression

In the Yogic tradition, the throat center is called the *vishuddha* that holds the meaning of creative energy. It vibrates with the color blue and is located in the throat region at the middle of the neck. It corresponds with the 5th energy layer of the aura, which is the astral layer. It corresponds with the thyroid gland and assist in circulating chi energy into the spine, throat, neck, esophagus and vocal cords.

This chakra holds the energy of wisdom and resonates with the primordial sound of OM, which expresses, harmonizes, and brings balance into your entire being. Energetically, a balanced throat chakra will result in clear communication, and appropriate self-expression. Its purpose is to assist in clear, creative communication both verbally, and audible forms. Sometimes, when there are blockages in the throat chakra people may show difficulty putting feelings into words or even have a fear of speaking. When this chakra is balanced well with sufficient chi energy flow, one is more likely to creatively express themselves and have health noted in the physical areas that this chakra energizes and nourishes, such as throat, esophagus, thyroid gland, vocal cords etc.

Visualize the blue throat chakra spinning in a clockwise direction while using the following affirmation. This will help keep the fifth chakra open and balanced:

"I love myself"

"I express myself with clarity and intent"

"I hear and speak truth"

"I allow creativity to throw through my voice"

"My voice is resonating with all others"

"My purpose in life is clear to me"

"I make wise conscious choices"

"I love myself"

Brow Chakra
The Perception center

Allowing in Intuition

The brow chakra is the sixth chakra and is called *ajna* in yogic tradition. The word ajna means to perceive and command. This is the center of vision and insight. It is often referred to as the third eye. It vibrates with the color deep indigo blue. This center is of much higher vibratory rate when compared to the lower charkas. From the heart chakra up, the chakras spin faster and are of more fine tuned subtle energies. This chakra is located in the middle of the forehead and is associated with the pituitary gland (master gland).

This chakra is connected to the sixth energy fields, which is called the celestial body, (which is an emotional aspect of the spiritual plane). The brow chakra helps circulate chi energy to enhance one's vision, insightful focus, psychic awareness and the ability to sense non-physical realities such as the aura. When this chakra is fully balanced, one is more aware of the environment and life path. When this chakra is balanced and flowing freely with chi energy, one may experience feelings of peaceful serenity, tranquility, and stillness. A balanced brow chakra also aids in insight and helps with clear vision and focus from a physical standpoint as well as a spiritual standpoint.

Visualize the brow chakra spinning clockwise with the color indigo. Use the following affirmation which will help keep this chakra open and balanced, allowing in chi energy.

"I love myself"

"My thoughts are clear and focused"

"I am one with my creator"

"I have clear vision on all levels"

"I am aware of my fine tuned insight"

"I am aware of my own sensitivity and the sensitivity of others"

" I love myself"

Crown chakra

Awareness center

Universal Unity

The crown chakra is the seventh chakra and it vibrates with the color light lavender. It is located in the middle of the top of the head at the Brahma Randha, where the fontanels are joined. It also holds the yogic name of *sahasrara,* which means awakening into the cosmic consciousness. It is connected to the seventh layer of the auric field, which is the Ketharic Template layer (also called the casual body). It energizes and nourishes the pineal gland, which is a small gland above the pituitary gland. The actual functioning of this gland is still under much research. Some researchers are finding this gland is helpful with the body's biorhythms and the timing of the onset of puberty and menopause. The crown chakra is associated with one's free will. The qualities of this energy center are associated with soul-consciousness and spirituality. In ancient writings, it is said that the great avatars that possessed spiritual mastership would have a halo or glow over this chakra and over the entire head.

When we pray for healing of any kind, chi energy in this chakra is vibrant and flowing.

Visualize this chakra with a light lavender color, spinning clockwise and feel the chi energy move in this clockwise fashion. Use the following affirmation to keep the crown chakra open and balanced.

"I love myself"

"I am at one with the universe"

"All are interconnected"

"I am at peace with my oneness"

"I am at peace with all of creation"

" I am one in body, mind, emotion and spirit"

"I love myself"

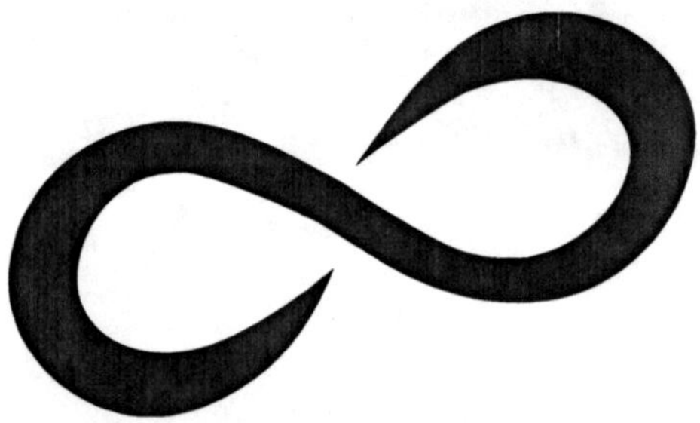

Meridians

The Bodies Energy Transportation System

The meridian system is the bodies energy transportation system. Traditional Chinese medicine for centuries has recognized this subtle energy system by which chi energy is circulated through the body. This circulatory system is referred to as channels or meridians. There are 12 main meridians in the body. Six of these are yang and six are of yin energy. Each one of these 12 meridians relate to all major organs, attempting to provide perfect balance, and homeostasis. There are two systems of channels or meridians, namely primary and secondary meridians. Primary meridians pass through internal organs but secondary do not. There are 12 pairs of primary meridians with chi flowing in continuous circulation through the following organs: lings, colon, stomach, spleen, heart, intestines, urinary bladder and liver. The primary meridians are named by the organ. They are connected to i.e. lung meridian, heart meridian. etc.

The yin and yang attempt to balance polarity in our meridians and entire energy system. Blockages or an imbalance in the Yin and Yang energy can occur in the meridians, inhibiting the proper flow of chi energy. Reiki helps to unblock and balance the meridians, restoring the healthy flow of chi (life force) energy.

To better visualize the concept of chi energy in the meridians, think of the meridians as a riverbed, which channels the water flow and irrigates the land, feeding, nourishing, and sustaining the substance through which it flows. In comparison to the circulatory system, it is like the blood flowing through the veins and arteries. The circulatory system moves blood around. The energy system on the other hand, moves energy through the meridians in order to provide universal chi energy to the tissues, cells and the entire body (bodies) Keeping in mind. I am not just referring to the physical body, but the emotional, mental, and spiritual bodies collectively. We are all one with this energy. We are holistic, multidimensional human beings - just beginning to understand there is more to" US" than just the physical body that we see with our human eyes.

Nadis

The nadis are somewhat like meridians in that they also are "channels". There is much Sanskrit detailed information on the subject of nadis but I will only address the basics due to the nature of this book. It is a part of the Energy system so needs to be addressed. A channel through which anything flows is actually a nadis. Included in this concept of nadis are acupuncture meridians, veins, and arteries of the cardiovascular system, lymphatic system streams, nerves, and muscles. Thus nadis can be translated as vessel, channel, cord, duct, or tube. There are two types of nadis. They are:

** SUBTLE nadis, which are invisible channels of subtle energy. (Such as meridians, Sushumna nadis, Ida nadis and Pingala nadis).
** GROSS nadis, which are channels of subtle energy visible as cords, vessels, or tubes (such as nerves or veins).

The subtle nadis are directly linked with the chakras. The Sushumna plays a major role in the energy system. These nadis do not take a physical form. The subtle nadis are connected to the autonomic nervous system. . There are 14 principle nadis. Of these, Ida, Pingala and Sushumna are considered the most important. Prana or chi travels from the pelvic plexus to the Brahma Randhra (the " cave of the *Brahman* which is the hollow space between the two hemispheres of the brain), and is situated in the interior of the cerebrospinal axis. The Muuladhara chakra (root) is the meeting place of the three main

nadis known as the Yukta Triveni. The Shumna originates in the root chakra and runs up the central spinal column. It branches into the Brahma Randhra, which externally this is the "soft spot" in a newborn infant that pulsates. After the first six months of life it begins to harden. Thereafter it can only be accessed through special practices such as Kriya and Kundalini yoga and others.

The ancient texts depict the chakras showing their major energy channels as figure eight patterns, flowingly wrapped around each of the seven major chakras. The two nadis, Ida and Pingala, which are polar opposites, masculine and feminine, begin at the first chakra (root) and end at the sixth chakra, polarizing and spinning each chakra. The sixth chakra is where dualities of consciousness and unconscious meet. The upper two chakras are associated with the realm of transcendent levels of consciousness.

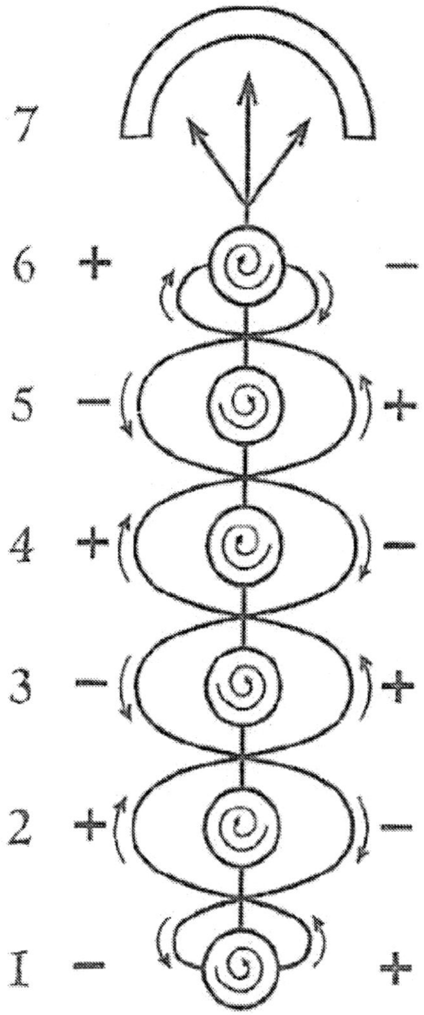

The Ida and Pingala ascend and descend in a spiral pattern, contributing to the chakras' spin. The Sushumna travels up the center.

Major Nadis

Chapter 3:

Reiki Touch and Energy Medicine

~~ Bringing it all together ~~

Your body is innately designed to heal itself. The ability of your body to maintain its health and overcome illness is among nature's most remarkable feats. You live in a physical world that systematically interferes with this natural capacity. Your conscious involvement in your health is required if you are truly interested in living a healthy, balanced and happy life.

It has always occurred to me, even as a youngster that we as humans must be made up of more than just material mass. I have always felt that we are complex creatures and there must be more to us than what meets the eye. As my life and spirituality have progressed, I now realize the concept of oneness. We are truly spiritual beings. We are breathing, living holistic entities consisting equally of physical, mental, emotional and spiritual bodies. We are more than just a brain, kidneys and lungs, heart etc. We are beings of light. We are spiritual, emotional and mental being as well. All of this forms and constructs the one being that we are. We are four bodies in one, making one holistic being.

It is vital to have an open mind when exploring the use of universal energy. In order to open our minds, we need to have the willingness to go beyond our everyday belief system and preconceived ideas. We need to incorporate a different view of ourselves. We are not mechanical robots but rather energetic beings. We need to honor all of the dimensions within ourselves and understand the great depth of our sensitive nature. To keep an open mind, one must be willing to examine his or her belief system and honor the holistic self.

Our minds act as filters for the bombarding stimuli, which enters our consciousness. Through Reiki Touch breathing techniques and practices, we can learn to tune into the "inner realms" of ourselves, enabling us to energetically connect with our inner oneness and center ourselves in the universal energy. We all have the ability to do this. We also have free will to choose the response to stimuli and stressors we are faced with. We are beginning to learn that we are unlimited co-creators of our own health. We have within us the capacity to create our lives the way we would like them to be. It is essential to have an understanding of life force energy, healing, and the need for our continued growth and development. Having an understanding of the energy system and the use of Reiki Touch can help us develop this awareness.

Personnel growth is a process, which sometimes includes physical or emotional discomfort. Growth and healing requires love and caring. It is love that nurtures, sustains and enhances life. We still experience pain in our lives at times, which allows us to go through the steps of our own journey towards true healing. Through opening our hearts, forgiving, and releasing emotion, we free unpleasant or negative energy from our beings. Sometimes this negative energy gets imbedded in our energy systems. We are all familiar with people who carry hatred, anger, or a negative attitude. They can be unpleasant to be around, leaving us feeling tired or drained of our own energy. On the other hand, it is a happy and joyous feeling when we are around people who radiate love and a positive attitude towards others. They let us see their inner joy, stability and peace. It is pleasurable to be around their energy. When ones' heart is open and free, the dynamic life force flows from the center of our being towards the outer layers of our oneness. Chakras and other areas of the energy system can become dysfunctional when they become congested or blocked by stagnant energy. They can become overcharged with unexpressed emotion. Dysfunction can occur at any level of our being, including yet not limited to, our physical being. One could develop a problem with circulation, inflammation, under or over functioning of a system or organ. On an emotional level, one may have low spirits, experience depression, anger or fear. Mentally one may experience rigid or negative attitudes, moodiness and even an inability to enjoy life. Transformation does not need to be harsh or dramatic. When we consciously choose change and healing, the process of growth begins. Working with the energy system is a gentle and unobtrusive way to guide us through release and eventual balancing, relaxation and healing. It is my hope that in working with Reiki Touch, you will become more aware of the healing and growth process, your own strengths, grace, beauty, and your own unique expression of life force energy.

BALANCE WITH REIKI TOUCH

A healthy life contains an even balance of the forces of Yin and Yang, which result in health of body, mind and spirit. The Yin (negative) and Yang (positive) reflect an energetic oscillation between polar opposites. Both are necessary to reach a balanced steady state of equilibrium within our dynamic bodies of constant change. The meridians distribute the subtle magnetic energies of chi, which provides the life force sustenance for all cellular structure and organs.

An imbalance in these polar energies causes a shift in the energetic equilibrium, which ultimately forms patterns of disharmony, imbalances, and illness. Energy dysfunction at the physical level may be reflected by imbalances in the energy system. An experienced energy practitioner using an accurate energy assessment can detect imbalances or blockages in the energy system.

Endorphins are released from the cells through the utilization of Reiki touch techniques for balancing and relaxation. Endorphins are polypeptides produced in the brain that acts as opiates that produce feelings of calmness and analgesia by binding to opiate receptor sites involved with pain perception. The therapeutic use of Reiki Touch enhances the release of endorphins into the blood stream, which provides a state of relaxation and balance. It is through this state of balance that our immune systems are enhanced, making it easier to fight off infection. It is also through a state of balance and relaxation, that the parasympathetic nervous system is able to take the lead, providing our cardiovascular systems with physiological homeostasis and clinically manifesting normal blood flow and vital signs within more normal limits. When endorphins are released, it's like taking a sedative; heart rate, blood pressure and respiratory rate all decrease, blood flows easily and naturally, thereby maintaining homeostatic mechanisms.

FACTORS "WITHIN" AND FACTORS "WITHOUT"

THAT AFFECT YOU

It is important to have an understanding of the factors, which have an impact on the health and well being of our energy system. Like any other system, we want to keep it clear, free of obstruction or imbalances. A healthy, free flowing energy system allows for a healthy individual. There are two basic factors that clearly affect your immediate field of energy and eventually the entire energy system. These are the factors <u>within</u> and the factors <u>without</u>. Imagine your immediate field of energy a little larger than arms length out from the physical body. This would be considered factors without. (Your total energy fields are much broader and are eventually affected as well).

We find it important to have clean blood and clean arteries. We find it important to have a balanced skeletal system and a healthy nervous system. The energy system also needs to be balanced, clear of blockages and healthy. Yes, the responsibility is on us. We have the free will to make the choices in our everyday lifestyle. By learning about the fundamental "FACTORS" within and without we gain the wisdom needed for health maintenance.

Factors from "within" are related to harmony or disharmony. What is comfortable for you may not be comfortable for another person, because we are all unique in our needs and comfort levels. Energies that play a role from "the factors from within" are thoughts of purity and love versus thoughts that are harmful or filled with fear, anger, hate and resentment. All thoughts and deeds should be positive or of a loving nature to ensure proper flow of the life force energy. The chakras will remain spinning and circulate chi energy with ease this way. This life force energy, discussed earlier constantly flows throughout our energy system to maintain balance and harmony. Remember also, the charkas, energy fields, meridians and nadias are all interrelated and affect each other much like any other system in our body. It's like a domino affect. Thoughts of dislike or irritation, fear, anger, mistrust, hate etc, all manifest a degree of chaos in your energy system and eventually can affect your health, your physical, emotional, mental or spiritual well-being.

Another more concrete substance that has a major affect on the "factors from within" are the types of foods and chemicals we come into contact with on a daily bases. The type of foods we ingest, the topicals and aerosols we are all exposed to, may include toxic chemicals. These preservatives and toxic chemicals can slow down and even block the life force energy thereby inhibiting the natural balance of the energy system. Our bodies are made to absorb and digest natural foods and plants from the earth. Our liver and kidneys are virtually ancient. They haven't changed any over the last several hundreds of years.

When unnatural substances enter our blood stream, our cells naturally put up a type of defense and reacts to un-natural preservatives or toxins as foreign material. Our organs are still prehistoric. They haven't changed as our food products and environment has. OUR ORGANS ARE NOT WILLING TO CHANGE WITH THE ENVIRONMENT. They expect and need pure organic foods and water in order to efficiently maintain health and homeostasis.

Kerlian photography is a type of photography that is highly sensitized and able to physically view bio-energy fields, including the aura of a person. During a viewing of Kerlian photography, which demonstrated people's auric fields, I was amazed with what I saw. It showed a viewing of a man eating a healthy, natural meal of organic salad, bread and fruit and a man eating a fast food meal including a hamburger and a soft drink. Their energy fields were observed to be completely different after they had started eating their meals. The man who was eating the fast food had a dark bluish-black asymmetrical, closed in aura and the other man, eating the healthy meal had a vibrant green, sky blue, well-developed, symmetrical auric field. This clearly indicated to me the impact of food products and the energetic affects of the energy system. The old saying may be right; "You are what you eat."

The substances listed below can and do play a role on the energy system. The more food additives and chemically altered foods we ingest, the lesser the energy system is able to balance, therefore altering its natural flow. This may result from absorption either by mouth or topically through the skin. This is only a very partial list of the substances that are known to be harmful to our body.

- Aspartame (an excitotoxin)
- High fructose corn syrup
- Monosodium glutamate (MSG)
- Hydrogenated oil or partially hydrogenated oil
- White sugar (better to use whole raw sugar)
- Dextrose, fructose, sucrose
- Palm oil
- Artificial color
- Splenda (Sucrulose)
- Soy protein Isolate
- Enriched white or wheat flour (better to use whole wheat)
- Mineral oil
- Petroleum products
- Pesticides
- Herbicides

The following is a list of food additives that are noted to be some of the **most harmful allergens** and poorly tested by the FDA for safety and many on this list are known to have carcinogenic affects.

- Ammonia
- Amyl alcohol
- Artemisia
- Aspartame
- Azo dyes
- BHA-7
- BHA- 7,40
- Blue No.1
- Blue No.2
- Boric Acid
- Bromated flour
- Bromated vegetable oil
- Butylated Hydroxyanisole
- Butylated hydroxytoluene
- BVO
- Citrus Red No.2
- Coal tar dyes-10
- Cyclamates-11
- Dichlorvos
- Erythrosine
- FD&C Blue No.1
- FD&C Blue No.1.1 Lake
- FD&C Blue No.2
- FD&C Blue No.2 Lake
- Formaldehyde
- Free glutamate
- Glutamates
- Green No.3

- Hydroxyethyl cellulose
- Indigo carmine
- MSG
- Ponceau 4R
- Potassium bisulfite
- Potassium metabisulfite
- Potassium prosulfite
- Potassium Sulfite
- Processed free glumanic acid
- Propyl gallate
- Sodium bisulfite
- Sodium cocoyl glutamate
- Sodium hydrosulfite
- Sodium metabisulfite
- Yellow No.6

(For further information refer to the references at the back of this book)

Try to get into the habit of reading food labels, aerosols, and other labels. If the ingredients are not listed, this is not a good sign. This seems to be much more prevalent in aerosols and topicals. This could be due to the fact that if the product is something you can ingest, they must, by federal law, indicate on the label the precise contents in the jar or container. More people are becoming aware of the harmful affects of what we put in or on our bodies. More and more, we are reaching out to whole food stores and farmers markets for a healthy food supply. Energetically we feel better if we eat fresh fruits and vegetables and fresh fish and poultry compared to a fast food meal loaded with a multitude of toxic preservatives.

There are many things that affect the " factors from without" Have you ever heard the saying " you are who you hang with?" Or have you heard "birds of a feather flock together?"

"Negativity breeds more negativity?" All of these clichés have some truth to them. Energies (including people) that you allow around your energy fields are considered to be "energies from without" because this is part of your environment. It is important to be aware of the energies of people that we come into contact with on a daily bases. When we allow negative people into our energy field, we are allowing depletion of our own energies, thereby diminishing our ability to balance, and well-being. It's much like allowing someone to sneeze in our face. We are likely to catch their germs and get sick. (There are however some energetic techniques that are protective against harmful energies, which you can learn about later). Select carefully who you allow into your energy field to avoid contaminating your own energy fields. We want a strong, healthy energetic stamina right? Then be around the right friends and people, and just as importantly, be in the right inner attitude as well. Keep in mind; the energy system has a direct affect on all the physical systems in the body. Remember, we are all connected in mind, body, emotion and spirit. They are not and cannot be separated. Please always keep this information in your frontal lobe. It's the key to understanding this entire book. All systems work systematically together as one to make us the one that we are. The FACTORS FROM WITHIN AND FACTORS FROM WITHOUT first and foremost affects our energy system. The energy system protects our outer shell and our entire being. THESE FACTORS affect the energy system FIRST, and then if disease or imbalanced energy is allowed to make its way through, eventually the other systems will be affected as well. Energy flows from the energy system and then branches out into the endocrine system, and finally reaching the other systems and organs.

Ideally, to live a healthy, balanced and happy life, one must be aware and exercise free will and discernment in allowing internal and external factors into our lives. These FACTORS play an integral part in the Yin / Yang balance within our total selves.

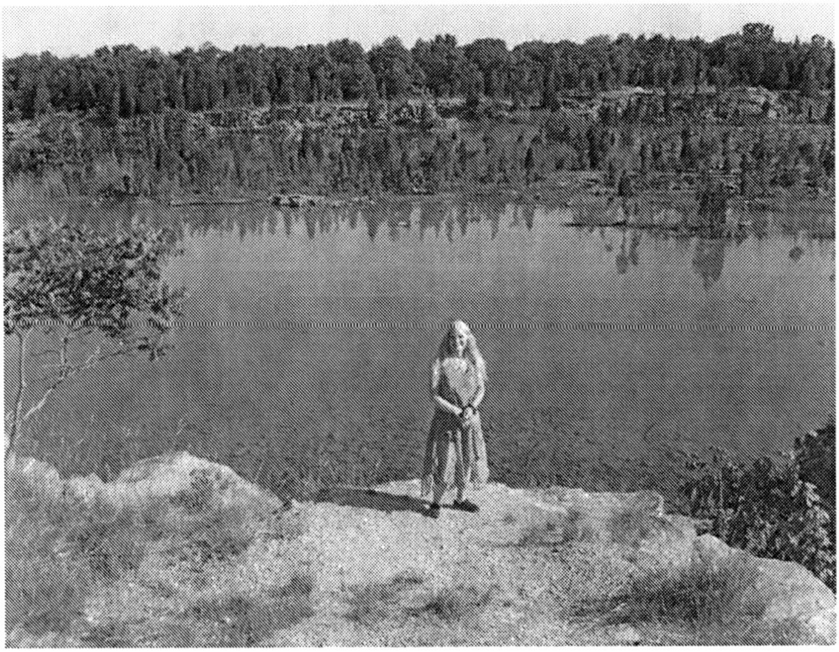

All Factors Affect Us

Chapter 4:

Reiki Touch Healing -

Practical application

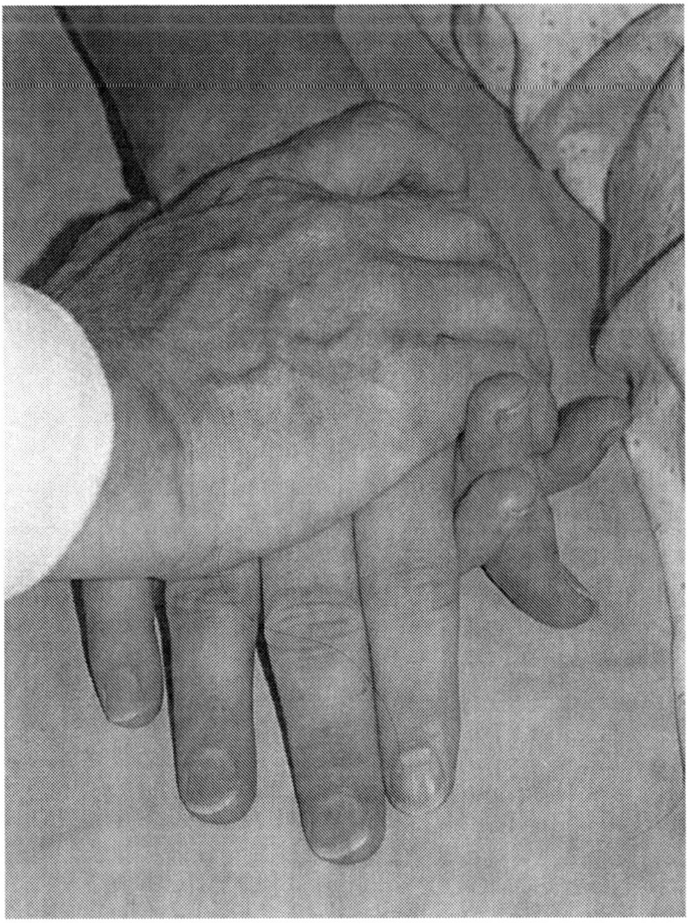

Healing Hands

The nurses' hands are inherently an instrument of healing. By using the word healing in this context, I am referring to interconnected healing of mind, body, spirit, and emotion. These bodies as mentioned previously are unified as one and cannot be separated. During Reiki Touch administration, the focus of the nurse is on that of balancing rather than the actual disease process of the patient or client. The ability to assist in the process of the therapeutic use of healing energy is inherent in all of us. This chapter is addressed to nurses because they provide frequent, important hands on care to the sick on a daily basis. The practice of Reiki Touch does involve opening oneself to a new mode or dimension of perceiving information. The practice of Reiki Touch is based on the concept of non-physical energy, which is a vitalizing universal force, which is always present and available for use. The practical use of Reiki Touch requires a conscious effort of the practitioner to draw upon the universal life energy and allow it to flow from the hands and into the patient, where it is needed for balancing, clearing, relaxation and healing. By reestablishing the natural flow of life energy in the patient, a sense of calm and healing will result. The practice of Reiki Touch involves making oneself an instrument for the healing force. This involves transformation of the practitioner, where you become "one" with what you have learned.

The Reiki Touch method not only helps relax and alleviate discomfort, but also tends to speed up the healing process. Sometimes a patient responds psychologically more than physically. You may hear patients claim at times, that they still have the pain but it doesn't bother them as much. They will rate the pain as a lesser degree on the pain scale. Reiki Touch is useful for both acute and chronic conditions. In general, patients with acute illness respond quicker than patients with a chronic condition. A patient with a chronic condition will probably require a longer time interval of Reiki Touch and may require it more frequently. When a person has been ill for many years, these disabling disease patterns become " in grained" or set in. For example the patient with chronic emphysema or with cancer may improve gradually over a period of time. On the other hand, in conditions of acute, emotional trauma or sudden acute pain, Reiki Touch seems to be more easily and readily absorbed with a more obvious therapeutic result noted.

Regardless of the acute or chronic condition, when Reiki Touch is used, a state of relaxation is generally observed. One way this method is able to bring about a more profound healing is through invoking a state of relaxation in which the individual is centered in the present moment. When relaxed, it becomes easier to diminish negative patterns of the past. During a Reiki Touch treatment, one can see the obvious signs of relaxation in the patient, such as slower and deeper breathing, decreased muscle tension, and dilation of peripheral blood vessels. This results in warmth of the extremities, pink skin, a lowering of the heart rate and blood pressure. These are indications that the method is effective.

Reiki Touch helps reduce anxiety. I have found it to be helpful not only with patients with stress-related physical disorders, such as tension headaches, high blood pressure and ulcers, but also those experiencing an emotional crisis or condition. Reiki Touch has a very calming affect on all these disorders. Words are not really necessary for treatment with Reiki Touch. Reiki Touch in itself can be a way of communicating with the terminally ill, who often are unable or too tired to speak. The terminally ill are very responsive to the process of Reiki Touch and greatly benefit from this modality.

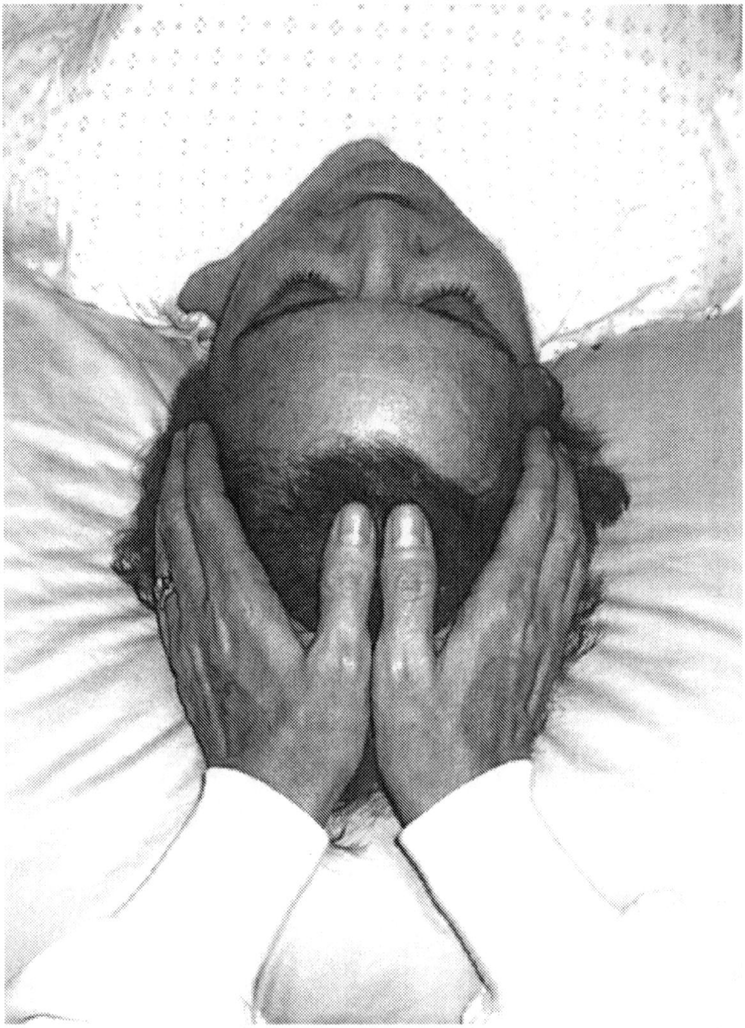

Reiki Touch

Cultivating the seed to become a powerful Reiki Touch practitioner has some requirements. These are compassion, self-discipline, and maintaining oneself as a clear, healthy channel. To be of good health, one must adhere to the principles of caring for the whole self. We must care for ourselves physically, mentally, emotionally and spiritually in a unified, balanced fashion. By living in a holistic manner, we are able to feel the benefits of well being and vibrant health.

By being compassionate, we have the ability to empathize with patients who are suffering. Being compassionate implies the desire to help without our own egotistical motives or personal gain. Compassion should never be confused with personal attachment. We need to be detached from the outcome. Self-discipline is necessary with Reiki Touch because it is a highly refined skill that is developed through regular practice. One can help people immediately after learning the basics, but with dedicated practice one's work and abilities become much deeper and more effective.

Some of the qualities of an effective Reiki Touch Practitioner include pure intent for healing, compassion, a positive attitude, self-discipline, a true desire to assist in the healing and well being of others and good health to ensure oneself as a clear channel.

This chapter, by no means takes the place of classes in Reiki Touch or formal training, however, I will highlight some of the essential concepts of Reiki Touch. When administering Reiki Touch, we touch our patients in a very non-intrusive, acceptable, professional manner. This is obvious because for one thing we are touching only in places on the physical body, which a nurse would normally touch. This is an important concept because it is an acceptable method for delivering the Life force energy in a natural manor. This is therapeutic not only in the eyes of the patients, but other staff members and family as well. When administering Reiki Touch one will be applying this "touch" to the forehead, head, shoulders, inner or outer elbows, wrists and hands. At times occasionally the ankles and feet are touched. When using Reiki Touch on your patients, it may actually appear so discreet that others around you may not even realize it is being done. If you are planning on doing a full treatment, ask the patient for permission after you have explained the use and benefits of Reiki Touch. Below is a partial list of some of the important concepts of becoming an effective Reiki Touch practitioner. It may take some time to become skillful with the following techniques, yet with practice, these skills will become second nature.

Focused breathing

Centering one's own energy.

Clearing one's mind

Pulling and releasing energy

Sending universal energy

Focused Breathing

By using focused breathing one is able to begin the relaxation and balancing process. In turn this aids in the ability to center and stay calm during the Reiki Touch session. The breaths need to have equal time given with both inspiration and exhalation. Beginners often use the four-count breath. You will inhale slowly to the count of four; then simply focus with intent on exhaling to the count of four. With some practice, this comes naturally. If you have trouble with focused breathing, practice it when you are alone a few times each day until you feel capable of using this technique in the presence of another.

Another effective breathing technique that works very well to center oneself is the three-second breathing technique. In this method, you will inhale to a count of three, hold the breath in to a count of three, and exhale to a count of three. Do this repeatedly from six to nine times or more, until you feel focused and centered. If you find with either of these methods, that your mind starts to wonder, just shift your thoughts again on the focused breathing. It takes some practice but it is very important to use one of these methods to learn how to relax and center yourself. If you know of another breathing method that works for you, that is also acceptable. The goal is to learn to center. The breath is the main tool you will develop in order to accomplish this.

Centering

Unless ones' energy system is in balance, he or she cannot effectively transfer energy to another. This is an important point to remember when doing energy work. To begin this process breathing and centering takes the lead. Centering is a very important technique one must have mastered in order to apply affective Reiki Touch to a client or patient. When I use the term "centering" I am referring to energetically being able to bring your inner strength and energy into your central channel. This is very balancing for the practitioner. It is through learning to energize and work with each one of the charkas starting with the root chakra and moving up mindfully to each next higher chakra, till we finally reach the crown chakra. Each time you focus on a different chakra, breath into it and visualize it spinning clockwise with the color related to that particular chakra. Don't move to the next chakra until you feel the balanced flow of the one you are working on at the time.

It is also good to ground your energy into the earth just prior to going to the next stage. Grounding is a part of centering. When one is properly grounded, there won't be a feeling of the energy being lost in space so to speak. One will feel clear, yet vibrant, and firmly rooted into the here and now. There are many different techniques available for grounding, yet one of the most widely used is with the use of guided imagery. Imagine yourself with roots of a tree under your feet and visualize these roots growing deeper and deeper into the earth. Slowly, visualize breathing into these roots. This technique is very helpful in grounding and in the continuation of the transference of energy with Reiki Touch. Centering means focusing on your own inner self and not allowing the outside environment to disturb you in any way. You will feel relaxed yet vibrant at the same time. Whenever you perform any kind of healing energy work, it is essential that you use grounding techniques before and after the work. It only takes a few seconds and there are many different grounding techniques available to learn. Regardless of the one you use, the main goal again, is to ground your energy, otherwise you may feel a sense of light-headedness and unable to perform other activities.

Clearing

Clearing your own thoughts may sound easier than it actually is. In order to do this, it takes a great deal of focused intent until you have mastered this stage. Focused intent becomes easier the more one practices it. You only need to clear or empty the mind of thought and chatter for a short time and think nothingness till the balancing process begins. By clearing the mind of outside thoughts, the universal energy can more effectively be used and flow easily. With enough practice, this entire process can be done in a matter of seconds. Focused breathing, centering, clearing ones own energy system and allowing yourself as a practitioner to become a clear vessel for the universal energy flow. Clearing actually sounds easier than it may be for you. You will want to keep your intent on the universal energy flowing, not other thoughts that may come into your mind. Keep in mind, you can perform Reiki Touch on a client in 30 seconds, or 10 minutes, depending on the amount of time you have available. An advanced one on one treatment may take 45 minutes to an hour. You learn how to shift your focus very rapidly in a way that best suits you and the patient, considering the environment and the work at hand.

Pulling and releasing energy - replacing with universal energy

When attuned to the Reiki energy, which must be done by an experienced certified Reiki Touch practitioner, your hands will have the ability to fully use the Reiki energy. You will be able to feel the imbalanced energy flow on the client. The practitioners' hands act as a tool to energetically pull unhealthy energy off and allow it to go through your hands and out to the atmosphere. This is all done in a mindful way and the practitioner may experience actual feelings of energy being pulled into the hands and arms. You may experience a variety of feelings in your hands as you begin to work with the energy. You may experience feelings of tingling, needles, warmth, coolness, heaviness, stickiness, emptiness etc. This negative energy is not really absorbed into the hands; rather, it is redirected into the universe for transformation. The goal here is to release blocked or stagnant, negative energy so that positive life force energy can be instilled within your clients energy system. It is important to dissipate the energy and not allow it to be absorbed into your own energy field. The clearing provides the space for complete renewal of universal energy to penetrate the subtle layer and the entire energy system of the client. The Reiki energy goes where it is needed most. The most important thing you need to remember is just to be there as a channel for the Reiki energy to flow. I, along with many other Reiki Touch Practitioners, believe one of the greatest effects from sending the Reiki energy is that when you give, you receive at the same time. In other words you get first dibs of the universal energy coming in. It flows into your own energy system first, then out of your hands, into the patients energy field and system, bringing about balance and feelings of peace, calm, joy and serenity that usually can not be put into words. An important concept to realize is that when the client is open to allow the energy in, it greatly increases the benefits of the treatment. It is also crucial to understand the vital importance of the nurse being a clear channel herself or himself in order to be the most effective for this kind of work.

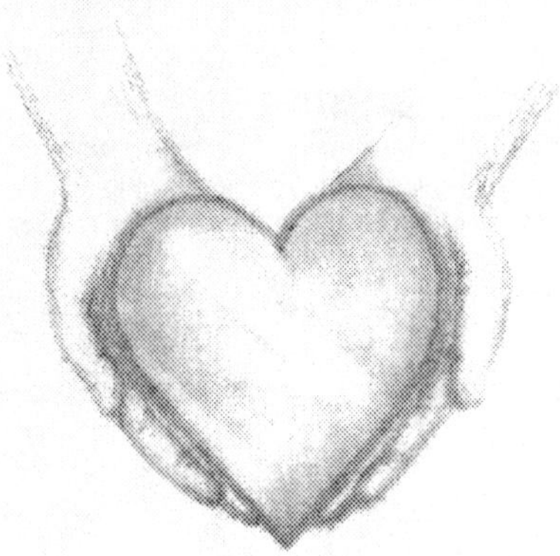

You will find, the more you practice using Reiki Touch, the more your hands will become sensitive to touch. You may experience feelings of tingling fingers, coolness, and feelings of warmth coming from the tips of your fingers. In fact, you may hear people ask you how your hands got so hot! Reiki Touch is never harmful and is always used for the clients highest good. Reiki Touch is a nursing intervention. Nurses are naturally touching patients, so why not amplify what you are already doing and provide calming, healing energy without using extra time. Remember, much energetic work can be done in just a few minutes. Patients use fewer narcotics and feel a greater sense of well being during Reiki Touch administration, not to mention there is a sense of trust and bonding that takes place with the administration of Reiki energy. When the patient feels better the nurses' job gets easier too. There is a heart-felt connection between the nurse and the patient. This is very therapeutic for the patient, especially if in a clinical environment, which often can feel uncomfortable. One can administer Reiki Touch during the bathing process or anytime the patient is experiencing distress, pain, anxiety or emotional upset of any sort. It is important to explain to the patient you are giving them relaxing Reiki touch, especially if they are alert and able to understand. On the same note, it is wonderful when the family realizes how helpful a soothing touch is. Families are more comfortable because they know their loved one is getting the best care.

I never believed touch therapy could have such powerful, dynamic affects on a person until I took my first class on energy healing over 12 years ago. I had read about it and actually just could not bring myself to believe it. It was after I learned to "feel" energy that the magical amazement in my healing journey began. Reiki Touch energy has made me the person I am today. Words cannot describe how it has affected me in total health, vitality, and balance. I know the old saying is "Seeing is believing", but with Reiki Energy, "feeling" is believing. It is very different than any of the other forms of energy healing because it is derived from Healing techniques of Japan, which stem back well over 5000 years ago. I think the best part about giving Reiki touch to your patients or clients is that it can be given to anyone with ease and acceptance.

Self-Healing

Unfortunately, it seems that nurses always put their own needs last. Focusing only on the care of the sick is not the most effective way to deliver the best quality care. When on the job, it is important to take a break and replenish yourself every four hours or so, even if just for a few minutes. Nurses frequently overlook lunches and breaks because they are so concerned their work won't get finished in a timely manner. They forget to be sharp; the brain needs replenished with nutrients. Keeping the physical body well nourished provides for a well balanced person all the way around.

Reiki Touch philosophy assists the professional nurse in developing keen insight into the needs of his or her individual needs and attitude, which plays an important role in the interrelationship between clients, family, and other caregivers. It is of utmost importance to stay healthy and vibrant, as a healing energy channel, in order to effectively meet the needs of the sick. A balanced life style encompasses the four bodies: mind, body, spirit, and emotion. Holistic healing means returning to a state of balance and harmony in ones life force energy. Self-healing can be used as a tool which should be used as a way of life. The tools should become habit in our daily lives.

Our bodies are attempting to maintain homeostasis every moment, weather we realize it consciously or not. Our own free will plays an important part in the self-healing process. If one of the four bodies is out of balance, it affects the other three naturally. In other words if your emotions or mental outlook is imbalanced, this may eventually have an affect on the spiritual and physical being as well. Some of the signs that one is in a state of imbalance are:

Physical ailments
Addictions – especially cigarettes and or alcohol or cocaine
Obesity
Depression
Moodiness, irritability
Malaise, complaining behavior, hysteria
Inability to focus, insomnia
Anger, fear, suppressed feelings
Suicidal thoughts
Inability to trust
Inability to care or form friendships
Undersexed or oversexed.

(There are many more. These are some of the most common ones.)

There are four universal phases of self-healing, and all hold equal value. Each of these phases can be as long or short lived as needed . Everyone's experience is individual.

The first stage is that of AWARENESS. If you don't realize there is an imbalance, you can't work on it. Pay attention to your own thoughts and deeds on a very conscious level. You may begin to question yourself as to why you said or did something. Pay attention to your feelings. If something triggers you into "feeling bad" stop and think about it or write it down and work on it later. Listening to our true inner self often holds the key to igniting the fire of self-healing. Actions of others in our lives and realizing the magnitude of your own thoughts and words play a very important role in the awareness phase. Only when we are fully aware of the problem or the imbalance, can we begin the healing process. If you see something on the list I have just mentioned, bring it in to your awareness and decide for yourself if you want to work on it or not. Another way to become aware of an imbalance is to listen to family, good friends, or the people in your life you trust. They love and care about your well being and won't steer you in the wrong direction. Hearing the same advice over and over from people that love you, surely could hold some weight. Also, by asking other trusted health care providers for their opinion is an option if you have any doubts in your mind as to whether a problem exists or not. Many imbalances are difficult for us to see, because we are " in" them so to speak. It becomes "habit" without really listening to your heart and you accept the imbalance as normal or acceptable. Other ways to recognize imbalances are through meditation, and learning to listen and feel what your inner guidance tells you. There is no wrong way to become aware. Once you are aware of the imbalance, fully embrace it on a conscious level. See it for exactly what it is, an imbalance within your being. You now have choice. Because you have free will, you can choose to stay in this phase indefinitely or move on to the next phase.

The second phase which is WILLINGNESS to change, involves some commitment. The second phase also involves duality. In this phase we can either accept the condition and weave our life around it, embracing it, or we can choose to be willing to change it. The choice is yours: accept it, or change it. Let me give you an example of making a healthy choice and exercising your free will to go into the phase of WILLINGNESS. A man has frequent coughing and visits his physician to finally get the testing needed to make the diagnosis of pneumonia. His physician tells him he needs to stop smoking in order to prevent diseases of the respiratory tract. The patient soon makes the conscious decision that he is WILLING to make a big change in his life and give up smoking. Each of us makes our own decision and there is no right or wrong in this phase. You have your own free will and no one can take your free will from you. This is a progressive process in which one moves through the four stages at a comfortable pace. One must feel comfortable prior to moving forward into the next phase. This second phase may take some time to mentally or emotionally adjust to. Take as much time as you need. We are all different in the amounts of time needed, but remember, one must go through all the stages and not skip any of them. You may need to learn to CARE about or to love yourself in this phase. Willingness stems from your own personal desire for change. Desire stems from your value system. If you value yourself then you love yourself. If you don't value or love yourself, you can learn to do this. This phase involves a commitment of making the conscious decision that YOU WANT TO CHANGE.

It is helpful to write your choices down or verbalize them to yourself, friends or loved ones. This makes your choice more concrete . " I have decided to give up cigarettes." Without completing this second phase one cannot move forward. True total healing of the four bodies comes from within and we must be the one to initiate it. No one can do this for us. Sometimes people become aware of an issue that needs to be healed, yet fail to follow through with the next phase. You can also blend your free will with Divine will and ask for help from your creator to allow you to make the change that is best for your highest good.

Seeking ASSISTANCE is the third phase of self-healing. In this phase, we seek to find an answer or path that will assist with healing the imbalance .You may need psychotherapy, energy based healing or traditional western medical modalities, or a combination of healing modalities. Reiki Touch healing, a type of energy healing often bypasses the conscious mind and goes to the root of the imbalance, which may be in the conscious mind or deep-seated emotions. The list of diverse avenues of assistance is endless. The important thing to keep in mind is, regardless of which modality your chose, follow through with it. Having a strong commitment in this phase will help you to stay focused and accomplish your goals. In this phase you will actively search for, and learn all the tools needed for healing or change to take place.

The forth and final stage is TRANSFORMATION, which integrates the tools learned in the previous step into your thinking, actions and your way of life. You have now taken on a new, fresh identity. You are more settled, secure, and comfortable within yourself and with your life. You have successfully adapted a new way of living, thinking, and acting, which is all part of the total healing process. Our total health is the most precious gift we posses. To keep it, we must always honor our total self. We must honor our emotions, our mental and spiritual selves, and our physical body, which is the temple of our true spirit.

There are occasionally times when people will go back and forth in the stages one through four. This is sometimes the case if the first strategy for change was not working. The important thing is to get the four steps going, be committed and aim towards living a healthy life.

Reiki Touch self healing and balancing

So far we have discussed Reiki Touch as a nursing intervention for the well being of the client or the ill patient. We have a clear understanding that Reiki Touch is useful for relaxation, pain control, and aids in general healing. This method may also be used for health enhancement for the nurse. Nurses give so much of themselves to others that they often put their own needs aside. One thing we must remember is the importance of balance. It is very beneficial to receive as much as it is to give. This is true from an energetic standpoint for all health care providers. Using Reiki Touch on oneself is an excellent way to balance, relax, and assist in your own self-healing. Reiki self-healing techniques are preformed by oneself, usually in a private setting. These techniques are done in any relaxed atmosphere where peace and calm are felt. It can be administered in your home or in a tub of water or a pool or lake. The practitioner can receive the same benefits that patients receive with Reiki Touch: relaxation, decreased pain and overall healing of mind, body and spirit. Through the Reiki Classes taught by a certified practitioner, you can learn these energetic techniques.

Once you are attuned to the Reiki energy you can use the techniques to bring stress relief, focus, and more clarity into your life with this powerful dynamic energetic healing technique .You will use the same steps in self healing that you will use in providing Reiki Touch to a client, such as breathing techniques, centering, clearing and allowing the energy to come in, to provide therapeutic affects. All you will need is an open mind, willingness to relax and allow the healing universal energy to work with you. By using the Reiki Touch technique on yourself, you will also have a deeper understanding of how it works on the patients you care for because you will have experienced it. Reiki Touch self-healing is extremely useful for balancing of the energy system, nervous system, and hormonal system. Through repeated use of this technique, you will be surprised at how you will grow as a person and how your life can change for the better.

As we move forward in time and progress with technology, we are beginning to realize that health care systems on a national level are beginning to implement many different complimentary therapies, including Reiki Touch. Even though this book's primary focus is on the use of universal energy for the patient or client, there is one other important point to be aware of. The universe is a dynamic, interconnected whole. All living organisms share the same life force energy and thus the principles of Reiki Touch have universal application.

In the next few stories I am about to share, I have changed the names to provide for privacy, yet these stories are true. I have had many more experiences, yet I feel it is important to share some of my favorites. The Reiki Touch benefits the patient and or families each time. I hope you find as much pleasure in reading these short stories as I have had in living and experiencing them.

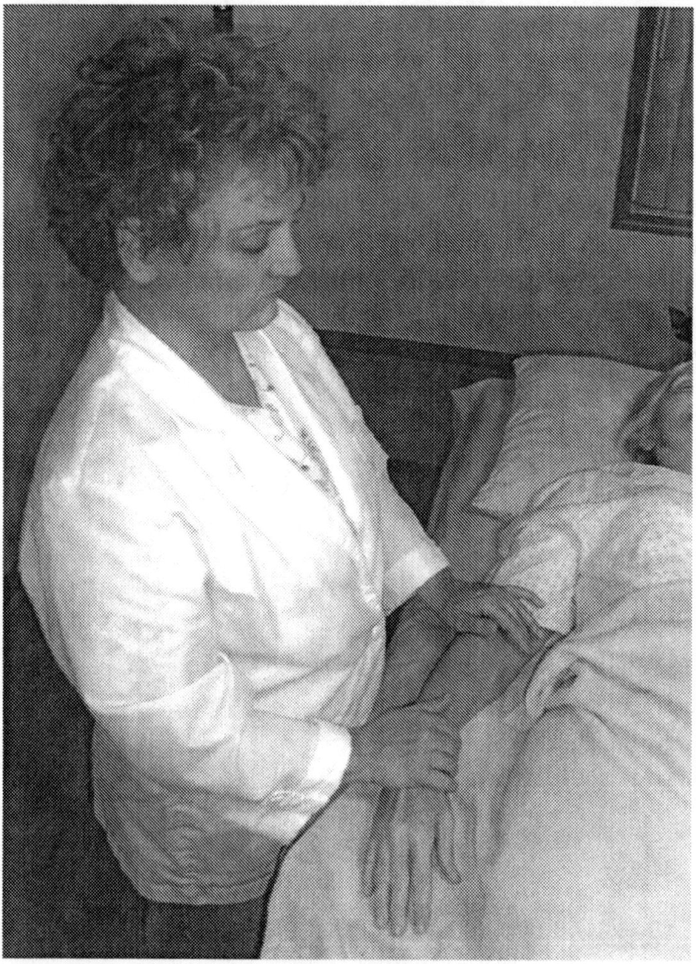

Reiki Touch for relaxation

Case # 1 ~~ The patient with a neurological disorder~~

" It's so hard to concentrate on what I am writing in my nurses notes about my patients", I thought, as I sat at the nurse's station in our very busy Intensive care unit. I could feel the irritable energy coming from both the patient and the nurse from bed space number 6. I began to wonder how all the "yelling" coming from that patient at frequent intervals was affecting the comfort of the other patients on the unit, not to mention other staff members including nurses and physicians. I felt beside myself as I heard occasional soft-spoken remarks from some of the other staff members….. "He's been like that" and " there is nothing we can do about it." As a Reiki Touch Practitioner, I know that Reiki touch can be very helpful for patients that are geriatric and for any kind of neurological disorder or insult. I spoke to the patients primary RN and made it known I was concerned. She and I discussed the patient's medications. "He can't have any sedation medications to help relax him because the Neurologist put all his sedatives on hold. He doesn't want to mask any symptoms." I could feel her frustration and exhaustion as she shuffled along to care for her second patient. As she hurried away the words remained in the air and directed to me, " Feel free to do some of your Reiki if you can, please". She was sincere yet in a hurry at the same time. I agreed to it with the nod of my head. As I entered the patient's room, I could "feel" his agony, despair, and irritability. I slowly and gently moved into his energy field. I began working with the energy intensely at about arms length because this is where I started to feel the heavy energy. I gently placed my hand with palm down on his forehead, then my left palm over his left inner elbow area. I had already initiated the controlled breathing and centering before even touching the patient. I began to use the Reiki energy. We connected energetically very quickly, yet in a calm and reassuring way. I almost felt like he was sucking me in. This is a feeling I get when the client or patient really is receptive to the energy work at hand. He lay there yelling and moaning at first but over a period of just about 3 to 5 minutes, I was able to reposition his head and remove his restraints. He was then snoring and fast asleep. I dimmed the lights as I was in a state of amazement because of the short time it took not only for the patient to stop yelling, but to also fall asleep. I quietly closed the sliding glass door. I made eye contact with the patients primary RN. She began to walk towards me with a bright smile. " He hasn't slept in over three days," she said as she walked closer to me. "I think that was his main problem," she added. A sense of relief filled the both of us, which lasted even after early morning hours.

It was about 6:30 am when the patient's primary medical physician stepped near the patient's room in bed space # 6. I happened to be standing close by. The physician gazed up at me with a baffled look on his face and said " What was he given for sleep last night? " I let him know about the profound affects from the Reiki Touch energy work I had experienced with him and that he'd been asleep ever since. His nurse came quickly around the corner as she left the other room and as she walked towards us said " He wasn't given anything other than a good dose of the touch therapy from Debbie" Needless to say, this was a win - win situation for everyone, the patient, nurses and other patients in our unit. The physician seemed very pleased. Reiki Touch doesn't always work this quickly and effectively, but in this particular patient it did. Many factors were involved with the outcome in this situation. At some level, the patient, even though not fully aware of his surroundings, was energetically open to the Reiki Touch energy. Touch, a nursing intervention, was needed and very effective for a patient that was unable to have sedation medications given to him because of a neurological disorder that was preexisting to his condition.

Case #2 ~~ The patient in respiratory distress~~

The nurses on our unit agreed we have great teamwork, especially when there is a crisis. This night, I found myself as a team player, yet in a surprisingly unexpected way. "One more medication" I said to myself. I only needed to pass one more sleeping pill and my patients' care would be completed for the evening till morning rounds. Even though I thought about this as I walked towards the back of our unit to retrieve the medications, I still had thoughts about the hours of charting I needed to catch up on. Another one of those very busy nights was taking place for me. "Oh well", I thought, "at least my two patients are stable". Just as that thought entered my mind I happened to see and "feel" something very peculiar practically pull me into room # 9, which was not far from my destination of the medication pyxis system. Quickly all my senses were involved as I could also hear this obviously distressed patient gasping for each breath of life as he slouched over in his bedside chair. I felt as if I had antennas extending out the top of my head and were straight up as I quickly yelled for help and rushed into the room. Without thinking about it, the Reiki Touch work began naturally. I'll never forget the helpless look in his eyes as if to say " I'm scared, please help me" I stepped behind this patient and thanked God one more time for making me a small person because of the obviously limited space in the room. I was able to reach the blood pressure machine for a reading with my left hand and held the patients shoulder with my right hand. The patient was terribly diaphoretic as I held him and began sending intense Reiki energy into his forehead and his shoulder. Another nurse came in and quickly handed me a moist washcloth for his face, as he was drenched in his own sweat. I laid this cloth on his forehead and continued to give the Reiki Touch through the cloth. It was very obvious to - now a crowded room that the patient was in acute respiratory distress and breathing rapidly at about 45 times a minute. He could barely talk and when he did, I encouraged him not to do so, in order to save his energy. I assured him with certainty in my voice as I made direct eye contact with him, my hands never leaving position, that he was going to be all right and we wouldn't leave him. The respiratory therapist entered the room and said she was going to put a mask on him because he was currently on 6 liters of nasal cannula oxygen and the patient refused. There was no talking him into anything and he made that very clear. I asked him if he could let us assist him back to his bed so we could start some important IV medications on him and get an EKG and he flat out said no! Here I am sending Reiki to a patient that can't breath and is not willing to go along with what we felt needed to be done. I spoke to the patient very slowly and calmly, instructing him to breathe slowly and to focus on relaxing into my hands. I felt the energy just kick in even stronger at about this time and I started noticing his breathing was slowing down a bit. His blood pressure, sky high at 210 over 110 with a heart rate of 140 wasn't what I'd wanted to see on the monitor. I continued the energy work as the nurses all hurried around me mixing up medications and getting the EKG machine ready for a picture of his heart. Within the next 30 to 60 seconds I noticed a dramatic change in his breathing. It had gone from 45 to 28 and now his heart rate was 120. Dr Wilber came in the room as I continued the work. He looked at me as if he was familiar with what I was doing. By this time, the other nurses had all left the room to gather supplies, leaving me there alone with the patient and Dr.Wilber, looked at me

asked, " Can you tell me about any of his lab results or how long he has been in distress?" I made eye contact with the doctor, continued to send the Reiki, and said with a soft voice "I don't know just how long he has been like this because I am not his primary RN, but I don't think it has been very long. His respirations have gone from 45 to about 28 over the last couple of minutes yet his lungs sound like they are filling up. If you would like, I will go check on his labs" Dr Wilber walked a little closer to the patient and myself and said with quickness in his voice "No, don't you leave him… he needs you more than you realize right now" The physician instructed the primary nurse to start an IV antiarrhythmic medication to slow the rate of his heart and to give some stat IV Lasix. The diaphoreses stopped by now and the breathing dropped to 22 breaths per minute, which is well within normal limits.
I continued with the work as the primary RN was opening the arterial line package via sterile technique. Dr Wilber said, as he started to pierce the patients skin at the area of his wrist, "now keep real still while I put this line in and consider yourself lucky to be calm enough to stay in that chair during an arterial line insertion." Later he told us that was a very rare for him to put an arterial line in when the patient is sitting up, yet was challenging forhim. After the line was inserted and sutured in place, the other nurses and I obtained a 12 lead EKG, still with the patient reclining in the chair. His heart rate was finally beginning to match the picture of a more controlled stable patient.

I made sure the patients call light was in reach as I knelt down beside him and now holding both his hands in mine, I said " Please know we are never far away and you can use this button to call if you need any help". He had a thankful look in his eyes and I could feel the heart connection between the two of us. Without words we both knew all was well for now and he had just gotten through a major crises. As I sat at the nurse's station to finally finish up my own charting, I was glad to exhale a sigh of relief.

Case # 3 Patient on life support and paralyzed

I was suctioning Mr. Jones mouth with the Yankauer suction device, as he lay there helpless after a recent stroke. I could feel the sadness in his heart. I sensed his fear and feelings of isolation, even though he was paralyzed and unable to verbalize or even make eye contact. He had been on the mechanical ventilator for about 3 days and nothing was changing or improving. His condition was very serious and sad because he was a fairly young adult. As I continued my care of brushing his teeth and suctioning, I naturally began sending him Reiki energy as a natural technique for relaxation. I could tell by his heart rate, which was slightly elevated that he was probably a bit anxious. One nice thing about administering Reiki Touch is that it can be given during other kinds of care. As I continued brushing his teeth, his wife entered the room. I introduced myself and explained to her about his mouth care when she came closer. "Has he had any visitors today yet?" she asked. "No", I stated, "just you to my knowledge but I have only been here for about 2 hours" Mrs. Jones had sincerity in her voice when she looked at me and said, " I get very offended at my in laws when they come up to visit because they are so negative. They sit right here in the room and talk about how bad this whole stroke thing is and how he probably will never walk again." She told me she wanted, and looked forward to him coming home. I reassured her that as soon as more information becomes available from his test results, we would notify her. She then asked me, "Do you think a persons negative or positive attitude affects the patient?" I assured her I had a very positive attitude about everything including life in general, which helped her feel at ease. She then asked me if I believed in Touch therapies. She smiled when I told her that was my specialty and that I was a Reiki Touch Practitioner. I felt the deep-hearted connection with Mrs. Jones as she revealed to me how glad she was that I would be giving Reiki Touch to her loved one. She asked me to teach her a few basic hand positions. I taught her some basic touch techniques that would benefit the patient and aid in his relaxation. So often we don't get to know the final outcome of our patients, but in the case , I was happy that she was so glad I taught her some basic touch techniques. The Reiki Touch not only allowed the patient to relax and be comfortable, but also brought about a sense of peace to his wife. It also gave her a positive way to express her love as she performs a helpful service. In this way, she is providing relaxation and care long after her husband leaves the hospital. Mrs. Jones was more than thankful for being given the education on such simple yet profoundly helpful techniques.

In this case the Reiki Touch administration provided a true sense of trust for the patients wife and helped provide a bonding for the patient and significant other.

Case # 4 ~~ Frozen shoulder~~

One of the most interesting experiences I've had was with Brenda, a middle aged woman suffering from a "frozen right shoulder". I cared for this client in my private therapy center rather then at the hospital. The interconnection of mind, body, spirit, and emotion was evident in this particular case. She had very little mobility in her right shoulder and hand. These areas of her body were very painful to even the slightest touch. I knew that when working with her I would need to be exceptionally careful when touching due to her intense sensitivity.

"I have been to numerous physicians and even physical therapy now and nothing is bringing me relief," she moaned, as she sat down on the Reiki table. After she laid down in a supine position, I assessed her entire energy system. Her chakras were balanced with the exception of about a 50 percent blockage in the solar plexus and 100 percent blockage noted in the right shoulder, right elbow and wrist. I began by clearing her energy fields, and continued the treatment as the very soft, relaxing music played in the mystical air. The room was filled with a sense of calm and lightness. It was a beautiful, intense, relaxing feeling that words really cannot describe. I then began the process of releasing the stagnant, blocked energy from the right shoulder and arm area. Sounds of release filled my ears as she lay there and began to cry. I encouraged her to let go and allowed her the time and space to ventilate her feelings through her tears. The crying was part of her release. Her emotional baggage she had been holding inside for so long was finally releasing through the Reiki Touch session. When I sensed it was time, I finished the treatment by filling the affected areas with universal energy. This treatment was obviously a very advanced form of Reiki Touch, unlike the basic Reiki Touch, which is preformed at a patient's bedside. I spent about an hour with Brenda while doing Reiki Touch. I then sealed and closed the energy and did the reassessment, finding all the chakras balanced and free of any imbalances or blockages.

As she sat up, I offered her a drink of water. I told her it was important to drink more water than usual to help rid of any toxins that had been released during the work. She yawned and said " Debbie, I feel so light and so different. I can't believe I was actually crying. It felt like something came over me and I just couldn't help myself." I gave her reassurance that it was ok to cry and that all sessions are held in strict confidentiality. She had nearly full range of motion in her shoulder and arm and her pain was completely gone. I spoke to her a couple months later and she stated the pain never came back and she was feeling just fine. This is a prime example of how the emotions had a huge impact on her physical well-being. Once she let go and allowed the emotional energy to release, her physical ailment subsided.

There are many more stories like these, some more basic yet some more amazing. Each Reiki Touch experience holds joy and value for the client as well as the practitioner. Reiki Touch allows me to feel in touch with my inner nature, which allows me to express my innate healing abilities.

Chapter 5:

Nurse as A Role Model Towards Holistic Health

Nurses are seen as powerful role models in that their health, behavior, and attitude are observed and taken to heart by the public eye. It is important that nurses be consciously aware of their presentation, and demonstrate compassion and professionalism in all aspects of care and communication. If nurses are healthy, well balanced, and positive, it presents a powerful message of actually walking their talk, and sets a good example for the patient to follow.

Now we will explore various aspects of how the mind, body, spirit, and emotion play an intricate role in the patients' perception of total health care. As mentioned earlier, these four bodies, united as one, bring about the essence of holism. The time is now for us to understand that our choices, voices and actions play a powerful role in the lives of our patients and in the everlasting value systems of other nurses to follow, for many years to come.

Nurses' Duties: 1887

In addition to caring for your 50 patients,
Each nurse will follow these regulations:

1 - Maintain an even temperature in your ward by bringing in a scuttle of coal for the day's business.

2 – Light is important to observe the patients condition. Each day fill the kerosene lamps, clean the chimney's and trim the wicks. Wash the windows once a week.

3 – Nurse's notes are important to the physician, so make your pens carefully. You can whittle the nibs to your liking, but the doctor must be able to read the notes.

4 – Each nurse on day duty will report every day at 7 a.m. and leave at 8 p.m., except on the Sabbath on which day you will be off from 12 noon to 2 p.m.

5 – Nurses in good standing will be given off an evening each week for courting purposes, 2 evenings if you go to church.

6 – Each nurse should lay aside from each pay a goodly sum of her earnings for her benefits during her declining years.

7 – The nurse who performs her labours and serves her doctors and patients without fault for 5 years will be given an increase of 5 cents a day.

8 – Any nurse who smokes, uses liquor, frequents dance halls, gets her hair done in a beauty shop will give the director of nurses' good reason to suspect her worth and integrity.

9 – Daily sweep and mop the floors of your ward, dust the patient's furniture and window sills.

Shelly McVimie 1906

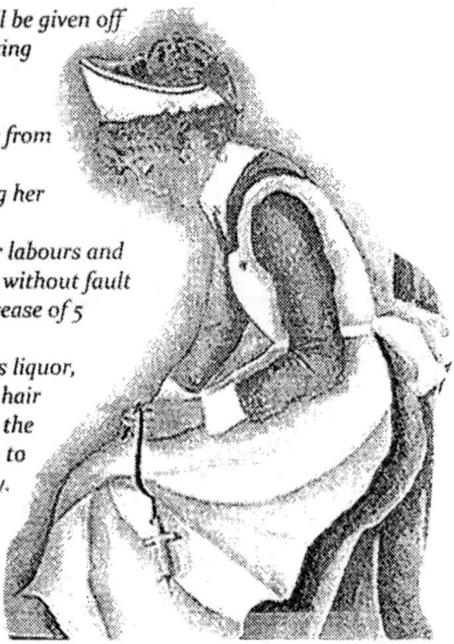

Figure 2: Nurses' Duties: 1887

We have choices every day regarding the attitude we will embrace. The impact of attitude and how people perceive us as nurses is very important. We cannot change the fact that people will react in certain ways. This is sometimes evident when caring for the sick. When people are sick, they are not always in the best moods. The best choice is to maintain a friendly, positive attitude, regardless of the situation at hand, or environmental circumstances.

I think we have all experienced being in an unpleasant environment due to someone's attitude. A negative or bold attitude speaks loudly and clearly to all others in the health care setting. It amplifies negativity and is uncomfortable in the health care environment. It can create a "**spreading of the energy**" effect. We as professional nurses, set the tone for a nurturing, peaceful, therapeutic, healing environment.

One evening while working on our busy the unit, I recall how the "spreading of energy" effect, started:

We were very busy in our nursing unit and were getting quite a few admissions at the same time. Our staff usually has a wonderful way of working together to make the admission process go smoothly for a new patient. I am very proud of our nursing unit because of this quality. I was preparing some medications for a critical patient we would be getting soon when I overheard Lucy, another RN talking at the nurses' station with a fairly loud tone of voice. " I've had it." She said, " I was not originally scheduled to be here but was marked on the schedule for twelve hours tonight. I'm constantly pushed around like this and am beginning to hate my job. Management just can't get it right. I was hired in for every other weekend and should have never been scheduled, not to mention I was shorted on my paycheck for the overtime I did last week. No one cares and it's just not fair."

I wondered how she had time to stand there and complain when all the other nurses were so terribly busy. As I continued to prepare the medications, Lucy's complaining was relentless. Soon, I noticed another nurse had jumped in on the conversation and she also started to complain about her job. Their voices were certainly loud enough for me to hear and I was standing about twelve yards away. The open doors of patients' rooms are much closer than that, so I knew they were getting an earful too. I've seen this sort of thing happen before and recognized the potential for it to infect the well being of other staff members and patients. I felt like I needed to do something. My knowledge of the concepts of Reiki Touch energy helped me intervene here.

I moved and stood close to Lucy while keeping my voice calm and respectful while directing my words to her as an individual. "Lucy, we can't help you right now and we are trying to take care of our patients." I said to her. " I'm not asking you to help me," she said, in a rather stern voice.

" Have you spoken to management about this concern yet?" I asked.

"Well of course not", she said. "They won't do a damn thing, we all know that!"

I looked at her frustrated eyes and said with sincerity, " I understand your frustrations, but none of us here can control your issues, and we can't change your circumstances. You need to tell someone who can help you." I was just being realistic, yet empathetic with her.

Her eyes seem to light up with passion "You sound like you are one of those people that work in management! Whose side are you on anyway?" she asked.

"I'm not on anyone's side," I said calmly. "When you signed up for this job at this hospital, did they tell you that there would never be any problems? You're wasting your energy by complaining about something that no one here can change. Please understand WE cannot do anything about it, so you need to tell somcone who can, and at a more appropriate time."

By this time her face was beet red and the other nurse who had lingered in the conversation had fled. Lucy decided reluctantly, to go about her business and the staff was able to get through the rest of the evening with ease and harmony.

Energetically, Lucy was "spreading" disharmony almost to the point of hysteria. I was able to energetically intervene for the sake of the patients and other staff members. Lucy had an issue and was frustrated about it, but rather than complaining about it uselessly, she needed to address it to the appropriate channel. It was not productive for anyone, including herself. We didn't need to be subjected to her mannerism. She was "spreading the energy" in an adverse way. Her "mind and emotion" was starting to connect to others. This could have eventually affected the "spirit" of the entire unit. The mind, body, spirit, and emotion all play an intricate role in the patient's perception of their health care. Later in the evening a couple of the nurses thanked me for intervening and talking to Lucy.

According to one large national survey in America, it was determined that the one profession, that the general public TRUSTS the most, is NURSES. We are labeled automatically by the public eye as a respected and trusting profession. Patients and family need to maintain that sense of trust to feel comfortable. Being friendly and kind to patients, families and other health care members is very important to the entire health care system. We all need to be very aware of our thoughts, actions and deeds in order to stay in a positive frame of mind, and display these qualities as a good role model in the public setting at all times.

Communication, that allows a patient to make choices, is rewarding to both the patient and health care provider. Little things mean a lot to a patient and they are very appreciative for the care we provide. Tasks, such as making sure the patient has enough water at the bedside, or that the call light is in reach, are just some of the things that nurses often take for granted. It is very helpful to ask the patient, just prior to leaving the room if they need anything else. This gives the patient a chance for communication, and therefore comfort. It also gives the patient a sense of control, which is something he feels like he has lost, now that he is unable to care for himself.

ATTITUDE

By Charles Swindoll

" The longer I live, The more
I realize the impact of attitude on life.
Attitude to me is more important than facts.
It is more important than the past, than education,
than money, than circumstances, than failures, than
successes, than what other people say or think or do. It
is more important than appearance, giftedness, or skill.
It will make or break a company.. a church….a home.
The remarkable thing is we have a choice everyday
regarding the attitude we will embrace for that day.
We cannot change our past…..we cannot change
the fact that people will act in a certain way.
We cannot change the inevitable. The
only thing we can do is play on
the one string we have, and
that is our attitude. I am
convinced that life
is 10 percent
of what
happens
to me and 90 percent how I react to it.
And so it is with you….
We are in charge of our attitudes."

The nurse's general health, appearance, and behavior play an important part in the perception of the patient. Nobody wants a nurse that looks like she just got out of bed. Of course it is much more pleasant to be cared for by a nurse with a nice clean, appropriate appearance and friendly disposition. It all comes down to practicing what you preach. Patients could also feel teased at times when they are on restricted diets and are exposed to the appearance and aromas of pizza, hamburgers, popcorn, and sweets. I am a little guilty of some of these things myself occasionally, but the fact still holds that there is always room for improvement and these issues need to be addressed.

One of the most common things nurses teach patients is their dietary needs and restrictions. I will never forget the patient that reminded all of us to practice what we preach.........

Bernice, a morbidly obese RN was sitting at her patients' bedside with some dietary paper instructions in her hands. Mr. Miller, her patient, had recently had a heart attack and was recovering quite well. I couldn't help overhearing the conversation due to the fact that our nurses' station is in such close proximity to the patients' room. Bernice instructed the patient as she sat next to him "You'll need to restrict yourself to about 2000 calories each day, Mr. Miller and avoid foods high in cholesterol. You are limited to a 2-gram sodium diet so you will need to choose foods with little salt and learn to not add salt to your foods."

Mr. Miller answered her, " And why do I need to follow these instructions?"

" Well, these instructions are standard for lowering cholesterol level and maintenance of proper weight and I want to ensure you receive good heart health education prior to your discharge, Mr. Miller. High cholesterol levels and obesity are two of the most common risk factors, which may lead to cardiovascular disorders and heart attack." She added. As I heard her speak, I thought how factual and correct she was, as the words gracefully flowed from her mouth, as if she had memorized it all. Suddenly I heard Mr. Miller perk up with a sharp voice and say:

"Have you had your heart attack yet? You look like you weigh over 350 lbs, so who are you to be preaching to me about diet?" At that point, she handed him the papers and ended the conversation. Mr. Miller may have been more accepting of this new life style change if the nurse herself had an appearance of good health.

The nurses' appearance and behavior has a direct effect on the patients' level of receptivity to education and information. Nearly 33% of American nurses are overweight in today's world. One of every 5 nurses has or has had a drug or alcohol problem and many nurses sadly have an addiction to cigarettes. Having these kinds of imbalances create an inability to function efficiently to provide the highest quality care available.

I recall another nurse, Deana, telling me of some of her experiences with secondary smoke. She happens to be allergic to many different things including smoke and perfumes, which can set off her asthma. She said that she is extremely sensitive to some of the inhalant chemicals, which included perfumes and the smell of smoke on someone's cloths and hair. At times just the brief smell of either of these could send her into an acute asthmatic attack. One evening she had a very valid complaint. She was telling me about one of our fellow co-worker nurses who had gone outside to smoke a cigarette on her break.

Deanna said by the time our co-worker retuned from break, she couldn't stand to be within more then 5 or 6 feet from her because the smell of smoke was so dreadful. She feared going into an acute asthmatic attack. She occasionally reacts the same way to perfumes that visitors and other health care providers wear. If a nurse can be affected like this, it stands to reason that patients and other people in general could have the same or similar reaction. At any rate, when I realized just how sensitive she is to smoke and other chemicals, I decided to completely stop wearing lotions and perfume.

How professional is it when a nurse walks into the patients' room smelling like an ashtray? I can understand how this could be upsetting to a patient. If the patient is a smoker it could make him more irritable by triggering a craving for a cigarette.

The most effective nurses present themselves as clean, appropriate in appearance with a smile and a friendly attitude. It is understandable, if we cannot maintain all these qualities all the time, but it is important to become aware of them. Nursing is a constant learning and improving process, and most of us do a pretty good job at it.

It's time we put the CARE back into health care. The art of caring includes compassion, touch, listening, emotional support and providing the best possible care for each patient as an individual. Things like compassion and spirituality are not actually taught in nursing school, yet most nurses go into the profession to express their compassionate selves and healing abilities outwardly. Please try to remember, above all else, that we decided to make nursing our profession because we care about people and want to make a difference. Therefore, one thing we should be focused on at all times, while at work, is our patient. This involves being aware and sensitive to how they feel and to their needs. The art of listening with a compassionate heart can provide great comfort to the patients and concerned family members as well. Often a patient feels so much better after they have vented their emotions. Just listening to a patient allows them to feel like some one cares. Another way of using your compassionate heart to offer emotional support and assist in the healing process is by using Reiki Touch during times of distress. A further way to provide comfort is to ensure the environment is quiet, especially during hours of sleep. Offer relaxation or soft music to aid in the healing environment. When a patient feels cared for, it is a natural tendency to feel more relaxed and secure, thereby quickening the overall healing process. When you feel better, you heal better because the emotional body affects the physical body. They are interconnected.

The art of touch includes spiritual touch, which can be very healing and beneficial to both the patient and nurse as well. One of these modalities is Reiki Touch, a form of spiritual healing and relaxation. The program of Reiki Touch for Nurses also teaches concepts of self-awareness, mind, body, spirit communication, clearing and healing modalities, which can benefit nurses and patients. Nurses can grow through self-awareness and self-healing techniques that are taught in this program. Reiki Touch is a comforting, compassionate touch that creates balance, healing, and a sense of trust, comfort and well being. Reiki Touch is different than other touch modalities in the fact that it is extremely user friendly. It can be administered with great ease. It can be easily administered in front of physicians, family, and other health care providers in the same environment. It is very noninvasive and acceptable by others. Reiki Touch provides relaxation, helps decrease pain and anxiety, helps aid in sleep, and provides general healing and an overall feeling of comfort. Reiki Touch only takes a few minutes and can easily be incorporated with other care. Reiki Touch is very useful for the patient and effective tool for self-healing and balance for the nurse. The art of using Reiki Touch encompasses the needs of Spirituality, compassion, and physical comfort in one modality. It is a way to give your patient that extra bond and reassurance that all is cared for.

~~ The mind, body, spirit and emotional aspects of care play an intricate role in the patients' total health ~~

Chapter 6:
How Do I learn Reiki Touch?
And commonly asked questions

Deciding to learn the methods of Reiki Touch through formal training is a professional decision only you can make. All of the Reiki Touch classes are full of fun, joy, and vital information on healing and practical use of this new energy touch therapy. Please check with the Center regarding contact hours (continuing educational units) for these classes.

Reiki Touch is a skill you will value and will have the rest of your life, adding much joy and healing to your life and the lives of others you care for. You may wish to take the first two levels to learn the basic methods of Reiki Touch and begin to use this wonderful modality on others. You may wish to take the advanced classes leading up to your final Master class. This will enable you to become a master practitioner, enabling you to have your own private practice if you wish. In a private practice, you are able to offer much more time and advanced skills of deeper energy for your client. If you are interested in attending or sponsoring a class in your area, please contact the Center.

The Reiki Touch Program is a multi-level program consisting of five levels of classes for formal training. The following is a brief overview of the multilevel classes available in order to become a Professional Reiki Touch Practitioner. After you have satisfactorily completed Level one, you can start using the Reiki Touch methods. Each level offers skills that are more advanced, therefore enhancing your skills. There are tests required at the end of each class, which require a score of at least 80 percent in order to continue on to the next level of training. The following classes offer contact hours for continuing educational units. Please check with the Center for details on current contact hours.

The International Center for Reiki Touch Training
C/O Debbie Glasgow RN
4990 Tawas Dr.
Ottawa Lake, Mi. 49267

Please refer to the web site for more information
phone number 734 888 2600
www.ReikiTouch.us
Reikiceu@aol.com

Introduction to "Reiki Touch for Nurses" For Stress and Pain Reduction

(for any of the following classes, check with the Center to find out how many contact hours are given for each class and further details or check the web site www.ReikiTouch.US)

In this class you will learn and receive:

- The complete history of Reiki including Reiki Touch and Traditional Usui Reiki.
- Knowledge of environmental stressors and ways to alleviate them
- Information between the relationship of stress and pain
- A complete definition of Reiki Touch and its use
- Information on the energy system including a clear understanding of Universal energy, the chakras, meridians, nadias, energy fields and their functions
- Vital information on the relationship between the Energy system and the Endocrine system and how this correlates with our health
- The experience active group meditation and learn how to center, use breathing techniques, guided imagery and affirmations
- Demonstration of the use of Universal energy and its role in reiki Touch for Nurses
- Professional Certificate ~ Introduction to Reiki Touch Therapy for Nurses for Stress and Pain Reduction ~ suitable for professional framing
- Contact hours for nurses

Reiki Touch for Nurses - Level One

In this class you will learn and receive:

- The interaction between the Energy system, the Circulatory and Nervous system, in relationship to our well-being, balance, homeostasis and total health.
- The process of how stress disrupts our health and ability to function at our highest capacity
- Skilled techniques used for assessing the energy system such as scanning and feeling different types of energy
- Experience of Reiki relaxation meditation and discuss the benefits as a group
- Practice with Reiki Touch self healing technique
- Practice with Reiki Touch using a partner
- The Level 1 Energy Attunement (receiving one Japanese Usui symbol)
- A professional certificate of~ Reiki Touch for Nurses-Level One ~completion and suitable for framing
- Contact hours for nurses

Reiki Touch for Nurses - Level Two

In this class you will learn and receive:

- In depth healing benefits of Reiki Touch
- Skills to assist in pain control
- The relationship between Reiki Touch and the release of endorphins (natural opiates)
- Mind, body, spiritual healing – interconnected concepts
- Therapeutic use of Reiki Touch with pre and post surgical patients and cardiovascular diseases
- Detailed information on the healing symbols
- The Level Two Energy attunement (including two Japanese Usui, and one Buddhist-Reiki Touch symbol)
- Hands on practice with a partner to use newly learned skills
- A professional certificate of ~ Reiki Touch for Nurses Level Two~ completion and suitable for framing
- Contact hours for nurses

Reiki Touch for Nurses – Advanced Practitioner Level

(There is a minimum of three weeks needed prior to taking the Advanced class after the Reiki Touch for Nurses - Level Two training)

In this class you will learn and receive:

- A description and hands on practice with the Richelle Reiki Touch Advanced Technique.
- Detailed information on two healing symbols – a Japanese symbol and a Hebrew- Reiki Touch symbol
- Advanced level energy attunement (including one Japanese Usui and one Hebrew- Reiki Touch symbol)
- Group Reiki Touch deep meditation for healing of self
- Practice sessions with a partner utilizing the Richelle Reiki Touch Technique
- A professional certificate of ~ Reiki Touch for Nurses Advanced Practitioner level ~ completion and suitable for framing
- Contact hours for nurses

Reiki Touch for Nurses - Master Practitioner Level

(It is important to have a full understanding of the specific requirements needed prior to taking this class. These are included at the bottom of this page)

In this class you will learn and receive:

- Advanced tools for healing and relaxation
- Detailed information on two Tibetan healing symbols
- A detailed discussion of values of the Reiki Touch Practitioner
- Information on developing your own practice
- Discuss other complimentary Eastern therapies and how they blend in with the use of Reiki Touch
- Reiki Touch Master Level Energy attunement (includes two Tibetan symbols)
- Practice time using Reiki Touch and Master skills taught in class
- The Ascension Healing Attunement
- Practice giving the Ascension Healing attunement to others
- Experience the Kwan Yin Goal Manifestation meditation in a group setting
- A Professional Certificate of ~ Reiki Touch for Nurses – Certified Master Reiki Touch Practitioner ~ completion and suitable for framing
- Contact hours for Nurses

It is very important to know that prior to signing up for this class the student must make contact with the instructor by phone or email to discuss details.

The concepts in the following article are very helpful for the Advanced or Master Reiki Touch practitioner in private practice.

Tools for a Healing Practice

By Debbie Glasgow RN, CRMI, CHTP

(Note: this article was published in "Beginnings" The AHNA Journal for Nurses)

You may have years of training and experiences. But no matter how talented you are as a practitioner, maintaining a successful practice requires a certain degree of professionalism and business etiquette. I am a nurse and a Holistic Practitioner with a well-established practice. Each week I see about 15 clients with issues ranging from depression to a multitude of physical ailments. Over the past ten years, I have gained a level of comfort and skill in my healing work that goes beyond mere technique or training. Whether you are a practitioner of massage, Traditional Reiki, Reiki Touch, Healing Touch or another healing modality, I would like to share these five basic concepts with you.

1. KEEP IT PROFESSIONAL

My healing space is neat and attractive in appearance without clutter. The sheets are always fresh, and the air smells clean and crisp. No eating is allowed in the room. I proudly display my professional Healing certificates in the room, so that clients can see that I have been well trained in the techniques used.

2. PROVIDE THE PROPER ENVIRONMENT.

Avoid outside noises and other annoyances from entering your healing space. Phones and beepers should be turned off, and lawn maintenance or mowing services should be scheduled around the hours of your practice. Generally, pets need to be taken out of the healing area because many clients are afraid of animals or even allergic to them. You also want to have the room set at the proper temperature. Prior to the start of treatments, I always ask clients to make me aware of any concerns they have regarding being to hot or too cold, not liking the music, or anything else they want changed. This open communication is very important and aids in developing a long lasting bond between your client and you. As a practitioner, dress professionally yet comfortably, avoiding tight clothes or low cut blouses that might show cleavage if you bend over. Jewelry should be minimal, if any. You may be different, but I find that even an ink pen in my pocket or a small ring on my finger can interfere with the energy flow.

3. CONFIDENTIALITY IS A MUST.

Always explain the kind of healing work you will be doing and be certain that the client completely understands the process. Make it a point to inform the client that anything said in the room, regarding assessment or findings that occur during the energy work, will never be discussed with another person. Also, reassure clients that their files will never be viewed by anyone but you, the practitioner. This helps build a sense of trust and sometimes encourages clients to feel free and open up and cry, or to discuss something else they may need to express.

4. LEARN THE ART OF SETTING LIMITS.

Your time is important. While each practitioner sets a different time limit, I generally give a one-hour treatment for a set price. Just prior to the treatment, I put on relaxing music. I know the music will last 50 minutes, after which I will have about ten minutes to reassess and ground the client. The 60-minute treatment is not ridged, but a basic guideline because I am dealing with real and sometimes-serious problems. Prior to a patient leaving, I take a moment to schedule his or her next treatment, asking that I be called at least 12 hours in advance in case of cancellation.

5. BE ACCEPTING AND NON-JUDGMENTAL OF THE CLIENT AND HIS OR HER DISEASE PROCESS AND/OR PROBLEMS.

Most importantly, be in the moment and provide your clients with the most professional, gentle and caring therapy that you know how to give. In addition, learn to disconnect from any outcomes that the therapy might provide. Each client's outcome is a part of his or her personal journey, and you do not need to take ownership. While you may offer words of empathy or kindness, know when you should occasionally refer a client to another holistic practitioner, such as a psychotherapist, if you feel it would benefit the client.

By following your inner guidance, developing good communication skills, and knowing how to set limits, you will add to the professionalisms and growth of your practice.

Commonly asked Questions

Is Reiki Touch just for Nurses?
Yes, at this time, Reiki Touch is offered to Nurses only. It is designed to be delivered at the patients' bedside or in a professional client/ practitioner setting. It is a therapeutic type of touch therapy for the sick. Even though it was technically designed for nurses and includes much scientific knowledge of the different body systems, the actual techniques could be taught to others with a true interest and intent to heal. At this time, however it is only offered to Nurses. Feel free to check with the Center for updated information.

Where can I learn more about Reiki Touch or take classes?
You can sign up for classes or obtain information or a brochure by contacting:
The International Center for Reiki Touch Training
C/O Debbie Glasgow RN
734 888 2600

Please refer to my web site for current address and phone number.

www.ReikiTouch.us

Reikiceu@aol.com

What other classes are offered at The International Center for Reiki Touch Training?
Reiki Touch For Nurses Intro through Master Level, Traditional Usui Reiki Classes from level one through Master training. There are also other various kinds of metaphysical classes taught at the center, such as Kwan Yin Meditation, Touch Reiki Yoga, Healing through Drumming, EFT, Metaphysical Science – levels 101, 102 and Advanced training, Eternal Flame Energy healing classes, Eternal Flame Consciousness classes. By 2009 we plan to also offer ***Certification in Metaphysical Science and Spirituality***, and with further training, ***Doctor of Metaphysical Science and Spirituality Certification.*** Please visit the web site or write the Center for more details.

How is Reiki Touch different from other types of Touch Healing Therapies?
Reiki Touch is very easy to administer and highly acceptable to physicians, families and patients because it is non-invasive when administered to the patient. It is very easy to administer in a public setting. It is acceptable to anyone watching it being administered. Unlike other types of touch healing, Reiki Touch deals only with touching very specific, appropriate parts of the body. Generally, the acceptable parts of the body to touch in a clinical setting are: the head, shoulders, arms, hands, ankles and occasionally the feet.

How does the Healing happen?
The practitioner acts as a channel, which allows the client to release old, blocked, congested or stagnant energy. Energetically, the practitioner works on balancing and releasing of blocks in the energy field. This allows life energy force to replace this negative energy for the clients highest good.

Can Reiki Touch be used with other healing modalities? Yes. It can be used in conjunction with massage therapy, spinal manipulation, or foot and hand reflexology and many others, depending on the clients' needs or circumstances.

Do the Reiki Touch classes offer contact hours for nurses? Yes, classes always provide for continuing educational units for nurses. It is important to contact the center for clarification on contact hours because specific number of contact hours may change from time to time.

What are the main therapeutic affects of Reiki Touch? The main affects of Reiki Touch are relaxation and pain and stress reduction, yet is also helpful with general healing for any condition. It is never harmful.

How is Reiki Touch different from Usui Reiki and Healing Touch?

The information, attunements and training for Reiki Touch includes all of the information and skills one would receive in Usui training program along with one Buddhists and one Hebrew symbol within the attunements. Other vital information and more advanced skills that deal specifically with patient care and the use of Reiki Touch by nurses are also included. While administering Reiki Touch, limited parts of the body are touched, such as hands, arms, neck and head and occasionally the feet. These parts of the physical body are deemed appropriate to touch in a health care setting. With Usui Reiki and Healing Touch a much larger portion of the body receives energy touch such as upper legs and trunk.

<u>What is the Reiki Touch attunement and why is it important?</u>

The Reiki Touch attunement is a standard part of the Reiki Touch education. You cannot learn Reiki Touch just by reading the book. You are required to receive the attunement, which ensures proper integration of the Reiki Touch energy from the instructor to the student via a special professional spiritually based ceremony. The attunement is very important because it is the means of ensuring that the student has the ability to have clear energy flow for the usage of this new energy. The attunement greatly enhances any practitioners' ability to perform touch healing modalities.

<u>How do the various levels of the Reiki Touch training differ?</u>

Levels Intro through level two are important because they teach you the skills necessary to be proficient in the delivery of Reiki Touch at the bedside. The more Advanced levels teach more technical advanced skills which would be useful towards one on one therapy with a client and practitioner such as in a private clinical setting.

<u>Why do the classes include Self Healing for the nurse?</u>

When the practitioner is energetically and physically balanced, the Reiki Touch energy flows more readily and is more easily administered to the patient. The Reiki Touch program encourages health on all levels for nurses because it is so important to maintain health in order to care for the sick.

References

Chapter One

1.) Gaynor,Steven. From Physician to Healer. Fla.: Center for Light, 2005.

Chapter Two

1.) Brennan, Barbara Ann. Hands of Light. N.Y.: Bantom, 1987.
2.) Gerber, Richard. Vibrational Medicine. SantaFe,N.M.: Bear and Company, 1988.

Chapter Three

1.) Wauters, Ambika. The Energy of the Chakras. Ca. : Crossing Press,Inc.,1993.
2.) White, Ruth. Using Your Chakras. M.A.: Red Wheel / Weiser, LLC, 2000.
3.) Farlow, Christina Hoza,D.C. Food Additives, A shoppers Guide To What's safe and What's Not.Ca. Kiss For health Publishing, 2004

Chapter Four

1.) Barnett, Libby. Reki Energy Medicine. Vermont : Healing Arts Press, 1996.
2.) Eden, Donna. Energy Medicine. N.Y. : Penguin Putman Inc., 1999.
3.) Hay, Louise. You can heal Your Life. Ca. : Hayhouse, Inc., 2005.

Chapter Five

1.) Chopra, Deepak, M.D. Quantum Healing. N.Y. Bantam Books, 1990.
2.) Judith, Anodea, PH.D. Eastern Body Western Mind. Ca.: Celestial Arts, 1996

Glossary

Attunement –A ceremonial initiation process that confers upon the recipient the ability to channel Reiki energy. The attunements involve sacred symbols. A Reiki Master performs attunements on students during training. In the Reiki Touch program, there is an attunement given to the students in levels one through master.

Aura- an energetic sheath that all living things are enveloped in. The aura or sheath is similar to the atmosphere, which surrounds and protects the earth. It is also referred to as the human energy field (HEF). The aura is a multi-layered sphere of energy that emanates from your physical body and interacts with the atmosphere around you. It is generally not visible by the human eye, yet easily visible by Kerlian photography. One can develop the ability to sense auras during the practice of Reiki Touch.

Centering –that of being consciously focused on relaxing your inner self and connecting to your higher self.

Chakra – Part of the energy system: also referred to as energy center (see energy center) The seven major chakras are the root, sacral, solar plexus, heart, throat, brow and crown chakra.

Endorphins – Opiate like substances released from the brain when our energy system is balanced and free flowing. Endorphins help induce feelings of euphoria, decreased pain and strengthening of the immune system.

Energy – inherent power, the capacity to do work, force of expression, Energy is constantly moving and changing and cannot be destroyed. Energy is a powerful resource that exists naturally everywhere and can be drawn upon to do work. One type of energy is universal energy, or life force energy. This energy can be guided and used by the practitioner to aid in relaxation, lessen pain and general healing.

Energy center – Chakras or vortexes of spinning energy within the human body. We mainly refer to the seven major energy centers when learning about energy healing. These energy centers are located along the spine from the perineum to just above he head. Each center holds a specific kind of energy.

Energy fields – (se aura) There are different layers of energy fields or auric fields. These layers are called subtle, emotional, mental, astral, and spiritual layers.

Energy system – An important system within all living things. It consists of energy fields, chakras, meridians, and nadis. Its function is to deliver, store and remove energy from the bodies.

HEF – Human energy fields, also called energy fields, or aura

Life force energy – Also referred to as Universal energy, prana, chi, ki, or life energy. Life force sustains all living things and all living things, without exception share in the generalized life force energy. This energy flows naturally in and around us through our energy system. In a state of health, life force energy flows freely in a balanced manner, nourishing all organs of the body.

Meditation – a state of being centered, focused, and calm in order to clear and open your energy system. It is a method of allowing you to receive higher levels of consciousness for guidance or awareness. A state of meditation may assist one in stress reduction, clarification, relaxation and balance the energy system to bring about a sense of peace and oneness.

Meridian –The part art of the energy system that deals with transportation of energy within the body. Chi energy or life force energy is circulated through the body through the circulating system called channels or meridians.

Nadis – a part of the energy system. All the channels in the body through which anything flows (including energy). There are two different kinds of nadis, which are called subtle nadis and gross nadis. The subtle nadis consist of meridians, Sushumna nadis, Ida nadis, and Pingalis nadis, which are all invisible channels for energy to flow. All subtle nadis are connected to the autonomic nervous system. The gross nadis are cords are cords containing subtle energy such as vessels, nerves, veins, muscles, and lymphatic system streams.

Reiki Touch – An energetic healing touch modality used mainly by nurses to help influence and restore harmony and balance within the energy system, which allows an alteration in the stress response and pain perception and assist in general healing These non-invasive touch techniques aid in relaxation and healing. The use of Reiki Touch alters stress response and pain perception and assists in general healing. Reiki Touch can be administered to a client in a clinical setting or private practice.

Spirituality – 1) of having to do with spirit or the path of our inner spirit or higher self
2) A dimension of higher consciousness that is connected to divine power and wisdom

Universal energy – (see life force energy)

Printed in the United States
115790LV00002B/78/A

9 781601 453273